How can 'Europe' be conceptualized under conditions of globalization? Going considerably beyond the more mainstream perspective of the 'European Union', this book series opens up a space for a variety of debates in relation to this question. These are consistently based on the agreement that it limits the analysis of Europe if we 'exotize' it by restricting it to itself. Consequently, Europe and its manifold aspects are contextualized and systematically linked to reference points in the global world or to the concept of globalization. This also means that 'globalization' loses much of the vagueness that it is often accompanied by, as it is repeatedly conceptualized and applied in relation to Europe. The series has a strong sociological and theoretical focus, but is open to interdisciplinary connections and various methodological approaches.

Europe in a Global Context

Series Editor

Anne Sophie Krossa
Fachbereich Soziale Arbeit
Katholische Hochschule Mainz
Mainz, Hessen, Germany

Marco Caselli • Jörg Dürrschmidt
John Eade
Editors

Migrants' (Im)mobilities in Three European Urban Contexts

Global Pandemic and Beyond

palgrave
macmillan

Editors
Marco Caselli
Dipartimento di Sociologia
Università Cattolica del Sacro Cuore
Milano, Italy

Jörg Dürrschmidt
Ludwigsburg University of Applied Sciences (HVF)
Ludwigsburg, Germany

John Eade
University of Roehampton
London, UK

ISSN 2947-8642 ISSN 2947-8650 (electronic)
Europe in a Global Context
ISBN 978-3-031-53772-1 ISBN 978-3-031-53773-8 (eBook)
https://doi.org/10.1007/978-3-031-53773-8

This Palgrave Macmillan imprint is published by the registered company Springer Nature Switzerland AG.
The registered company address is: Gewerbestrasse 11, 6330 Cham, Switzerland

Paper in this product is recyclable.

Acknowledgements

This volume presents the main results emerging from the research project "State Capacity and the Capacity to Aspire—the Corona pandemic as a testing ground of local migrant integration: Stuttgart, London and Milan", funded by the Volkswagen Foundation under the "Corona crisis and beyond" programme. Jörg Dürrschmidt, Professor at University of Applied Sciences (Public Management and Finance) in Ludwigsburg, has coordinated the overall project, which includes the research team at University of Roehampton in London, led by Professor John Eade, and the team at Università Cattolica del Sacro Cuore in Milan, led by Professor Marco Caselli.

First of all, we would like to thank all the people who actively took part in the research process, namely, the authors of the chapters in this volume as well as Michal Garapich, Markus Rutsche, and Alessia Rambelli. We are also grateful to Volkswagen Foundation and its staff for the economic and administrative support, which made this project possible.

Heartfelt thanks go to all the "experts" and "non-experts" who have either been interviewed or whom we encountered during our field research, for having shared with us their stories, ideas, fears, dreams, and suggestions.

Finally, we would like to express a special thanks to Anne Sophie Krossa, editor of the "Europe in a Global Context" series which hosts this volume, the entire staff at Palgrave Macmillan and Springer Nature, particularly Sharla Plant, Liam Inscoe-Jones, and Arun Prasath, as well as Nasima Begum and Vinitha Jayabalan at Straive, whose professionalism has been essential to the publishing of this volume.

Contents

Notes on Contributors

Marco Caselli is Professor of Sociology and Methodology of Social Research at the Università Cattolica del Sacro Cuore, Milan, where he also holds the role of Director of the University Centre for International Solidarity. From 2017 to 2021 he was Coordinator of RN15 "Global, Transnational and Cosmopolitan Sociology" at ESA (European Sociological Association). His publications include *Trying to Measure Globalization. Experiences, Critical Issues and Perspectives* (Springer 2012) and with Guia Gilardoni (Eds) *Globalization, Supranational Dynamics and Local Experiences* (Palgrave 2018).

Jörg Dürrschmidt is Professor of Sociology at the University of Applied Sciences (Public Administration & Finance) Ludwigsburg, Germany, where he is also co-director of the affiliated Institute for Applied Research (IAF). Between 2006 and 2009 he acted as "European Outreach Officer" of the GSA (Global Studies Association, UK). Previous publications with Palgrave include: (2007) (with Graham Taylor) *Globalization, Modernity and Social Change: Hotspots of Transition* and (2019) (with York Kautt) (eds) *Globalized Eating Cultures: Mediation and Mediatization.*

John Eade is Professor of Sociology and Anthropology at the University of Roehampton, Visiting Professor at Toronto University, and former Executive Director of CRONEM (Centre for Research on Nationalism, Ethnicity and Multiculturalism), which linked Roehampton and the University of Surrey. After research in Kolkata (Calcutta) on the social identity of the educated Bengali Muslim middle class, he completed his

PhD in 1986 on Bangladeshi community politics in Tower Hamlets. Since then he has researched the Islamisation of urban space, globalisation and the global city, British Bangladeshi identity politics, and travel and pilgrimage. His publications include the single authored *The Politics of Community: The Bangladeshi Community in East London* (1989) and *Placing London: From Imperial Capital to Global City* (2000), the single edited *Living the Global City* (1997), and the co-edited *Transnational Ties* (2008), *Accession and Migration: Changing Policy, Society, and Culture in an Enlarged Europe* (2009), *The Ethnically Diverse City* (2011), and *Reliving the Global City: Global/Local Processes* (2018).

Silvia Malacarne is a PhD student in Sociology, Organizations, Cultures at the Università Cattolica del Sacro Cuore, Milan, where she also collaborates with the University Centre for International Solidarity. A Teaching Fellow in Sociology of Cooperation and in General Sociology, she works on mutual learning in the context of development partnerships.

Shamea Y. Mia After obtaining her PhD in Sociology from Goldsmiths College, University of London, in 2015, she has held a number of research and teaching positions at the University of Suffolk, the University of Greenwich, Queen Mary, University of London, the University of Warwick, and the University of Roehampton. She has worked on projects on identity and belonging, children and schools, mental health and inequalities, health and access to care, South Asian (mainly Bangladeshi) diasporas and social systems. She teaches and researches at the University of Roehampton.

Samuele Davide Molli is a post-doc researcher at the University of Milan (SPS Department) and received a PhD in Sociology in 2020 from the Università Cattolica del Sacro Cuore (Milan) with a thesis on the relation between religion and migration. He is involved in a research project which focuses on the religious citizenship of immigrants and investigates the new religious pluralism generated by migration to Italy and its social and civic implications. He has also undertaken research on discrimination in collaboration with ASGI—Association for Juridical Studies on Immigration—and the development of postmodern forms of volunteering in the field of homelessness and social marginality.

List of Figures

CHAPTER 1

Introduction: State Capacity, Capacity to Aspire and Layered Resilience During a Pandemic

Marco Caselli, Jörg Dürrschmidt, and John Eade

1.1 A Research Project on the Impact of the Pandemic

The COVID-19 pandemic, which began to manifest itself in the last months of 2019 and then spread to the whole world in 2020, was an event in its own way unique in human history. It was undoubtedly an epochal fact of global significance in various ways. It affected all areas of the globe

M. Caselli (✉)
Dipartimento di Sociologia, Università Cattolica del Sacro Cuore, Milano, Italy
e-mail: marco.caselli@unicatt.it

J. Dürrschmidt
Ludwigsburg University of Applied Sciences (HVF), Ludwigsburg, Germany
e-mail: joerg.duerrschmidt@hs-ludwigsburg.de

J. Eade
University of Roehampton, London, UK
e-mail: J.Eade@roehampton.ac.uk

M. Caselli et al. (eds.), *Migrants' (Im)mobilities in Three European Urban Contexts*, Europe in a Global Context,
https://doi.org/10.1007/978-3-031-53773-8_1

and, thereby, stimulated collaborations all over the world that attempted to deal with the emergency, even if these collaborations were only partially satisfactory in terms of results, particularly in the scientific and political fields (Holley, 2020; Apuzzo & Kirkpatrick, 2020). Furthermore, the pandemic will probably have a lasting impact, especially on some patterns of everyday life and ways of looking at the world and the future (Furceri et al., 2022; Rodríguez-Caballero & Vera-Valdés, 2020).

However, this undoubtedly global phenomenon has shown its most significant and dramatic impact at the national and local level (Davvetas et al., 2022). Numerous and diverse strategies have been implemented to try to contain and deal with the pandemic across the world by both national and local authorities, by civil society organizations and ordinary citizens. Even within the same local context, the ways of experiencing and dealing with the pandemic have differed from institution to institution, from neighbourhood to neighbourhood, from family to family and from person to person (Ogueji et al., 2022; Clement et al., 2023).

The pandemic has, therefore, proved to be a profoundly ambivalent event, as is typical of many global phenomena and of globalization itself. Although the pandemic was a profound challenge for all humanity, at the same time it brought out and emphasized the differences between people, territories, institutions and other collective actors. Looking at its effects on people, it can be said that while we have all been directly or indirectly affected by the pandemic, its impact has been very diverse, just as the resources that people could mobilize are different. Consequently, the ways in which people have reacted to the pandemic itself have also varied.

Because the pandemic was for everyone an experience that was, in many respects, unexpected—even if not unpredictable—none of us were adequately prepared. It required everyone—individuals, institutions and other collective actors—to make a considerable effort to deal with its impact—an effort most of the various actors were unable to accomplish on their own. Given the effort required, the core question that our research has sought to answer here is the following: where do people with a migration background look for help and orientation in times of a societal crisis?

This is not a trivial question, given the 'habitual indeterminacy' (McGhee et al., 2017) of their positioning in society. Typically, people become acquainted with the institutions and culture of the society of settlement while simultaneously maintaining some links with their countries of origin. This 'double process of socialization' may, under favourable conditions, foster the development of innovative hybrid identities but, under less favourable conditions, it might instead trigger marginalization tendencies in both the country of settlement and the country of origin. While we would agree that under normal circumstances the second generation is the 'litmus test' (Penninx & Garcés-Mascareñas, 2016, p. 19) in this balancing act, a societal crisis might serve as a more profound and accelerating laboratory of social migrant integration.

We claim in this volume that the Corona pandemic is indeed such a crisis which has unveiled the ambivalent societal positioning of migrant populations. Those with a migration background are overrepresented as 'key workers' in jobs that were crucial during the pandemic, such as health care, public and domestic cleaning, hospitality and other services, postal and other delivery jobs, as well as crucial assembly line work. In other words, the types of jobs they undertook made it possible for others, mostly members of majority populations, to work safely from home. However, it is precisely through these jobs that people with a migration background have been at higher risk of COVID-19 infection and transmission, making them an easy subject of public opinion scapegoating (OECD, 2020). This, in turn, indicates an ambivalence in the 'spaces of solidarity' that emerged during the pandemic. On the one hand, 'effective residence' fosters a sense of pragmatic solidarity between members of the majority populations and those with a migration background—or, in any case, those with a cultural background different from that of the majority. On the other hand, behind the debate about resources available for public health, there lurks the difference between solidarity and belonging (Triandafyllidou, 2020).

Against this general background, our volume draws on results emerging from a comparative qualitative study of people with a migration background in Stuttgart, London and Milan. It seeks to understand how the pandemic has affected institutional trust, networks of solidarity and feelings of belonging amongst Turks in Stuttgart, Bangladeshis in London and Peruvians in Milan. It should be noted here that the terms used to describe people with a migrant background differ in each of the three contexts. Among Bangladeshis in London, members of the third or even fourth generation have spent their entire lives on British soil and therefore cannot be labelled as migrants. Categories used in British public and academic discourse have changed over time to reflect these changes—from 'black' to 'Black and Ethnic Minorities', 'Black and Minority Ethnic', 'racial and ethnic minorities' to 'minority ethnic', and recently also those with a particular 'heritage'. Likewise, in Germany and Stuttgart, there are now four generations of people with a Turkish migration background. Some of them have indeed been born in Turkey, some have been born in Germany, some are German citizens, some have Turkish or dual citizenship, some see themselves as dedicated Muslims, while others follow Islam as a cultural tradition. Processes of individualization and differentiation make it less plausible to talk of a 'Turkish community' or 'migrant community' for that matter. Instead, there are various 'milieux' based on socio-economic positioning as well as cultural values amongst those with a Turkish migration background. It is only a matter of convenience when subsequently we fall back on terms such as the 'Turkish migrant community'. In the Italian context, on the other hand, the situation is rather different, since Italy has a much more recent history as a country of immigration, and a significant third and fourth generation, for example, has yet to emerge. Consequently, the use of the term 'migrants' appears decidedly more appropriate in this context. Therefore, when we use the terms 'migrants' and 'migrant populations' in this volume, we are not necessarily referring to people who have had a personal experience of migration, but to those whose family roots and, at least in part, their identity refer to their country of origin rather than to where they are currently living.

Our study seeks, then, to better understand how those from different migrant backgrounds have reacted to the pandemic socially, culturally and institutionally. We started from the assumption that while normally the position of migrant communities is associated with unequal access to generally scarce societal resources, such as wealth, power and social prestige, the Corona pandemic shifted the focus to more specific variables: living in segmented or overcrowded conditions, working in jobs with higher risk exposure, facing difficulties with online schooling due to a lack of appropriate electronic devices and encountering barriers to accessing health care and information due to linguistic, legal and administrative constraints (migrationdataportal.org). Accordingly, outreach programmes towards migrant communities have already been initiated by the WHO, the EU and national governments in particular. At the same time, the cultural resilience of minorities may also play a key role. Consequently, our focus in this project is not on statistical evidence that describes migrant communities as marginalized groups further left behind by the Corona pandemic, but as survivors who can mobilize moral and social resources that other groups in Western society might not possess to the same extent—such as dense family ties, embeddedness in transnational networks and the routine of a religiously structured everyday life supported by a cluster of agile community organizations.

In order to explore the complementary dynamics of migrant integration during an extraordinary societal situation, we focus on two concepts: 'state capacity' and the 'capacity to aspire'. The first refers to the capacity of governments to enforce rules and deliver services across a variety of functions, levels and communities. This depends less on the body of law and more on trust in the professionalism of administrative staff, on the reliability of public institutions and on convincing leadership. It could be argued that state capacity especially appears during times of crisis, such as this pandemic (Fukuyama, 2020). However, state capacity is relational in character since it also relies on the self-organizing capacity of the underlying society. Appadurai (2013) has aptly referred to this as the 'capacity to aspire'. It describes people's efforts to maintain everyday life routine and to change the future from a neutral space-time into a vision of the 'good life' worth pursuing. However, the Archimedean point of the argument is the development of a sociological understanding of 'layered resilience', thereby adapting a concept so far largely used in ecological research (Obrist et al., 2010; Hidalgo et al., 2021), in order to uncover the middle ground between state capacity and the capacity to aspire.

1.2 From Heroism to Normality—Placing the Concept of Layered Resilience

The issue of resilience has been central to understanding modern society in the twenty-first century. We only have to recall its fundamentally reflexive character as analysed in Ulrich Beck's study of 'risk society' (Beck, 1992). More recently, Elliott and Turner (2012) have aptly called for an investigation into the potentials of an 'elastic society' that could absorb the challenges posed by 'new catastrophism'. These challenges the authors see as emerging from the limits of a neoliberal globalization in general, and in particular brought about by 'global civil instability' and 'global disease from HIV to SARS and H1N1' (ibid., p. 157f., 165f., 171). Accordingly, long before the Corona pandemic struck, there was already a 'ubiquity of resilience' in the sense of 'patterned adjustment adopted by a society or an individual in the face of endogenous or exogenous shocks—across the broad social science spectrum' (Bourbeau, 2015, p. 1958).

Indeed, resilience has developed into a buzz word that has moved from ecology, health and psychology into education, family science as well as urban and regional planning. Hence, it could be argued that the concept has itself become more robust or resilient. While it was developed within individual-oriented psychology, it became a sociological concept applied to various social groups and sub-systems such as the family, neighbourhood, city and region. Two aspects of this development are of particular importance for the argument pursued in this book. On the one hand, emphasis has shifted from deficit orientation towards strength orientation in the analysis of resilience. While the deficiency approach is best exemplified by the 'superkid' who roly-poly-like bounces back despite detrimental circumstances in the family environment, the strength-based approach focusses on the potential for growth emerging from the inter-individual or systemic coping capacity. Accordingly, the key to robust resilience is the inter-individual effort to maintain a problem-solving 'normality' of everyday life amidst stresses and challenges rather than individual personality factors. We could summarize this as a relational rather than an actor-centred understanding of resilience (Black & Lobo, 2008; Maurović et al., 2020, pp. 338–341; Mu, 2021). Accordingly, resilience as a societal capacity can only be understood, when it is seen as a capacity evolving between state and non-state actors. Moreover, and drawing on the work of Penninx et al. (2020/2004, p. 8), we would describe resilience as the outcome of two intersecting processes: the 'top down' provision of 'opportunity structures' by state institutions, on the one hand, and the 'bottom up' mobilization of civil society initiatives in order to 'activate' these opportunity structures to reflect their own interests (see Fig. 1.1 as modelled on these thoughts).

Sociologizing the concept of resilience has also fostered sensitivity towards the difference between passive 'adaptation' and active 'adjustment'. It became clear that adaptive resilience could actually help to perpetuate detrimental circumstances, whereas adjustive resilience could carry an element of transformation and resistance (Mu, 2021, pp. 16–17; Maurović et al., 2020, p. 339).

While Bourbeau suggests that until recently 'migration scholars have been relatively absent from this vibrant discussion' on resilience (2015, p. 1958), migrant families have often exemplified the shift of emphasis in this debate. A specific type of 'family cohesion' is something we routinely associate with migrant families and ethnic groups, often specified with reference to 'family ethnicity', that links the individual members of the family with collective identification, kin relations and daily rituals and practice (Black & Lobo, 2008, p. 36f.). This, in turn, is often seen as the

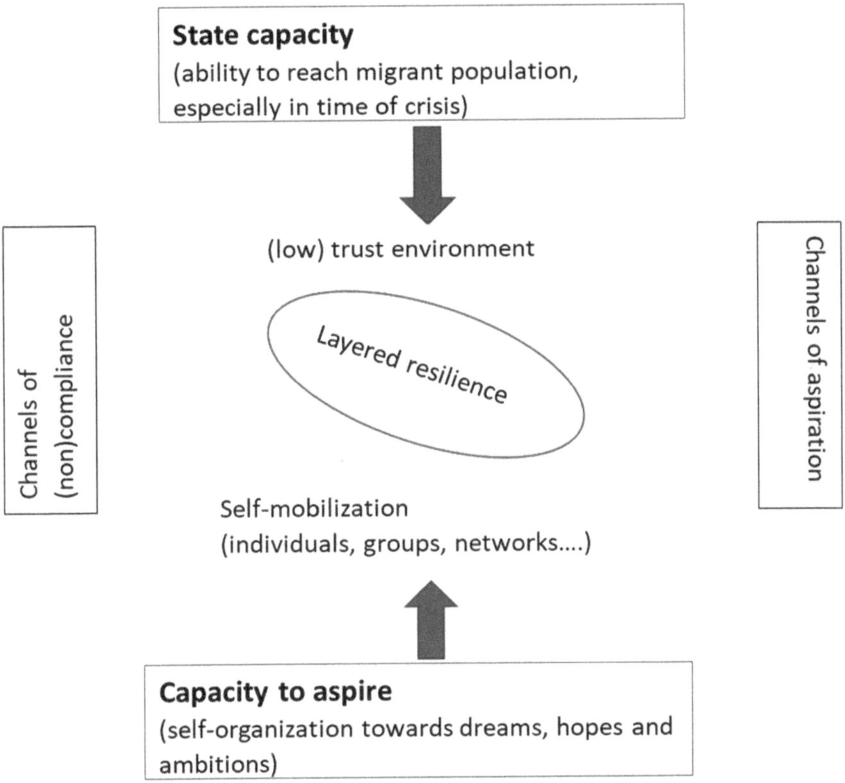

Fig. 1.1 The place for layered resilience

basis of typical 'migrant optimism' that helps to explain the 'immigrant paradox' according to which migrants, carried by high life ambition in general and educational aspirations in particular, tend to overlook disadvantages in terms of resources and are therefore prone to seeing the glass half full rather than empty. However, at the same time it becomes clear that this 'immigrant paradox' relates to numerous factors at various levels, such as attitude to work and education, language skills, active ethnic heritage, obligation to kinship and community, (non)discrimination in the education system and the overall acculturation gap (Doty, 2016; Bermudez & Mancini, 2013).

1.3 Solidarity and Belonging—Social Cohesion in Times of Pandemic

The COVID-19 pandemic is an amplifier, but not a game changer in matters of integration and integration policy. It has in a rather experimental fashion revealed basic tendencies of cohesion and exclusion which are prevalent in all modern societies that rely on migration. As already emphasized above, lockdowns and quarantines fostered a sense of humanistic solidarity based on 'effective residence' (Triandafyllidou, 2020, p. 1). Even if based on privatized compliance, it extended to all members of society. It could be described as an ad hoc solidarity based on the democratic socialization of risk and risk perception, as well as the sense of mutual obligation following from that. The prolonging of the pandemic, however, increasingly placed questions of 'public health' above humanitarian concern and thus reemphasized the nexus between belonging and solidarity (ibid.). This effectively reasserted the supremacy of national community and the rescaling of institutionalized welfare across the difference between citizens, temporary residents and visitors, reminding those hovering on the margins of irregularity about their limited entitlements to long-term care and protection. The resulting asymmetries with regard to access to pandemic-relevant information and knowledge, health care services, and (home) schooling might have raised public awareness and concern—but at the same time, it displayed nothing but the well-known Janus-faced character of the modern state: on the one hand, a 'liberal-democratic state' committed to mobility and universal human rights, while, on the other hand, a 'nation state' with its particularistic tendency towards an exclusive collectivity (Joppke, 2004, p. 452).

This paradoxical logic of pandemic inclusion should, in turn, refocus our attention to at least two other aspects of social integration. Both further support our argument that what we observe in the wake of the pandemic is not something exceptionally new but, instead, follows a certain path-dependency. On the one hand, there is a growing awareness that cities as social and political entities might be following a distinct or 'intrinsic logic' of development, which leads them to pursue a more liberal mode of integration and integration policy. There is indeed a long-standing debate about the decoupling of urban from national citizenship, based on the self-confident statement that even or especially during the upheavals of globalization, 'place remains fundamental to the problems of membership to society' and that cities are therefore particularly 'privileged sites for the current negotiations of citizenship' (Holsten & Appadurai, 1996, p. 188f.). Various authors have, therefore, started to link the creeping emancipation of 'substantive citizenship' (in terms of access to civil, economic and cultural rights based on exercised residency) from its complement of 'formal citizenship' (in terms of legal status given by state law) (ibid., p. 190) to the difference between nation-state-based 'citizenship' and urban 'city-zenship' (Bauböck & Orgad, 2020).

This development ties in with the impact of European multi-level governance on migration and integration governance and policy. Intense policy-uploading and downloading between the EU, national and regional-cum-municipal levels has led to changes in the realm of integration politics and policy too. Accordingly, it has been argued that sub-state political units have become more empowered and involved in migration policy, in general, and migrant integration policies, in particular (Hepburn & Zapata-Barrero, 2014, p. 4). Whether this amounts to a sustainable 'local turn' in migrant integration policy—with benefits for the societal standing of migrant communities—remains open for debate (Schönwälder, 2020, p. 3). What a view across the diversity of local migrant integration in Europe, including the UK, Germany and Italy, over the last couple of years suggests, at any rate, is a general tendency away from multiculturalism towards more assimilationist policies with an emphasis on civic integration. This has partly to do with a change of societal climate after 9/11 and also with neoliberal austerity politics in the name of the mainstreaming of public services (Galandini et al., 2019; Campomori & Caponio, 2017; Green, 2007).

If there is indeed such a 'national turn on local integration policy' as suggested by some observers (Emilsson, 2015, p. 2), this is not to be equated with homogenization and not just because cities are by their urban nature counterpoints to cultural homogeneity. This is why we follow the assumption that 'minor contextual differences' such as administrative structure, migration history, civil society tradition and urban leadership can make a difference in terms of local social cohesion (Vertovec, 2020, p. 24). It is these contextual differences that we will further explore in the following chapters of this book.

1.4 A Note on Methodology: Comparative Sociological Forensics

There is good reason to investigate the relationship between state capacity and the capacity to aspire at the local level. It is at the municipal level where a great deal of public services for migrants are offered and where actual integration policy occurs (Garcés-Mascareñas & Penninx, 2016). On the other hand, migrant communities' complex (non)engagement with the surrounding society also evolves through a local prism of values, tradition, communication and dissent (Glick Schiller & Çağlar, 2011). Accordingly, we can draw on research that has investigated the diversity in local political practice in relation to migrant minorities (Schönwälder, 2020) or indeed has already attempted to investigate the interplay between integration policies 'from above' and immigrant self-organization 'from below' (Penninx et al., 2020/2004)—through a pioneering comparative European study at the city level.[1]

At the same time, we do not want to align our argument with an 'epidemiological sociology' interested in the 'social shaping of population health' (Link, 2008). Following health trends and understanding the link between health disparities and issues of social status and ethnicity is part of the project but we focus on the role played by institutional trust, everyday life routine and identity in coming to terms with the pandemic. Therefore, our approach is perhaps closer to an emerging 'critical-interpretative medical anthropology' (Rivera et al., 2019) that combines 'structural competence' with cultural understanding. This approach refuses to 'blame the victim' for health disparities and emphasizes that vulnerabilities are 'racialized and gendered and citizenshipped in multiple ways' (ibid., p. 3). Our approach also stresses the importance of the 'social world', in which and by which people come to terms with vulnerabilities and health disparities.

In terms of methodology, then, we find our study best described as a 'synchronic multiple linear' comparison (Lucassen, 2004), since it follows two or more migrant groups in different local contexts over the same time period. The three interrelated local case studies bring together an innovative combination of single- and multi-sited ethnography (Gielis, 2011). We seek, thereby, to use the local contexts of three areas within the

[1] We are not aware of a comparative European study that has explicitly focused on this emerging field of 'middle ground resilience' towards a crisis event, in general, or a pandemic, in particular.

European region which have experienced the pandemic differently, in order to sharpen the tool of 'minimizing and maximizing difference' for analytic purposes.

The Turkish (Stuttgart) and Bangladeshi (London) migrant communities provide an excellent initial contrasting perspective. On the one hand, they are both 'settled migrant minorities' (largely 'born here') and precisely for this reason, especially in the English public debate, as we have already noted, these communities are often described as 'ethnic minorities' or 'migrant ethnic groups' more often than 'migrants'. On the other hand, Bangladeshi Muslims have an additional post-colonial link to Britain in contrast to the purely utilitarian and still latent framing of the Turks in Germany as 'guest workers'. This difference is demonstrated by access to citizenship and an official recognition of Islam as a religious identity. The Milan case broadens the analytic perspective in two distinct ways. Peruvians have arrived relatively recently since Italy became a destination for international migrants only in the 1990s. At the same time, they come from a Catholic-majority country and have settled within a Catholic-majority country. Church affiliation can provide a key resource for playing out questions of un/belonging and this strengthens our comparison, since we will be considering the use of mosques and churches, different religious and community representatives and different/similar ways in which people themselves view what is going on.

In order to reconstruct the interplay of state capacity and the capacity to aspire, we have mainly relied on semi-structured Corona lockdown interviews with municipal and religious officials, political and community activists ('experts') as well as 'ordinary' residents ('non-experts'). In other words, on the one hand, we wanted to meet those who, given their position and their role within the realities under study, were privileged witnesses of the dynamics to be analysed and particularly possessed information that was relevant for the study. On the other hand, we also wanted to listen directly to those who were not involved in local positions of authority and experienced the pandemic in everyday life.

Given the particular context in which we conducted our research, some of the interviews had to be conducted online via Skype, Webex or Zoom. We did not consider this to be an inferior way of qualitative interviewing but we did remain alert to both continuity and difference (Johnson et al., 2021). We interviewed 13 people in Stuttgart (5 'experts' and 8 'non-experts'), 17 in Milan (11 'experts' and 6 'non-experts') and 15 in London (10 'experts' and 5 'non-experts'). Our fieldwork was enriched by ethnographic observation of some of the developments affecting the migrant communities we studied, specifically in religious contexts, as soon as restrictions on movement were lifted.

In detail, for the study of Bangladeshi in London, John Eade and his colleague, Michal Garapich, decided to conduct the research in Tower Hamlets in the following way. The first stage ran from March to August 2021 when they focused on collecting secondary data, recruiting respondents and making a number of visits to the borough. The team leader, John Eade, had been working closely for many years with Michal Garapich at the University of Roehampton through their mutual interest in the study of migration and ethnicity in London and had published several papers together (2009a, 2009b; Drinkwater et al., 2008). John Eade also was well acquainted with the Bangladeshi community in the area, since he had been involved in various academic and community projects there since the early 1980s (see Eade, 1989, 1997a, 1997b, 2007, 2013).

For the second stage, which began in September 2021 and ended during December 2022, they recruited a British Bangladeshi post-doctoral research assistant, Shamea Mia, to undertake and transcribe interviews with ten 'experts' and five 'non-experts'. John Eade continued to visit the borough to sit in on some of the interviews, meet other Bangladeshi colleagues and see how the area was recovering from the economic and social disruption caused by the pandemic. Shamea Mia interviewed the ten 'experts' between September and December 2021 and again during the summer of 2022. They were embedded in a variety of community organizations—mosques, neighbourhood and community centres, the NHS and the local council—and were skilled at mediating between Bangladeshi residents and public bodies. Four of the ten were heavily involved in local community organizations, while the other six consisted of a borough councillor, who was also a youth worker, a doctor who was also a social influencer, a Covid Champion who was also a businessman, a Bangladeshi Hindu legal adviser who worked at the Bangladesh Welfare Association on Brick Lane, an imam at the Brick Lane Mosque next door, a journalist at a local Bengali language TV and radio station and a funeral director. Eight were male and two female, most were fluent in at least two languages (Bengali and English), while seven could also speak Sylheti—a Bengali dialect used by most Bangladeshis since the vast proportion of migrants had come from this north-east district of Bangladesh. Of the five 'non-experts', two were female university students, whom Shamea met at the East London Mosque, while three had migrated from Italy—a male caretaker at the Brick Lane mosque, whose brother lived in Sicily and his wife and children in Bangladesh, and two female homemakers who had migrated from Italy with their husbands and children.

Jörg Dürrschmidt and his colleague, Markus Rutsche, conducted the research in Stuttgart. We followed the classic sequence of qualitative interviewing, starting with 'pilot cases', followed by a brief period of 'snowballing', before turning to a more purpose-driven 'analytic sampling' of cases. Behind what sociology calls 'cases' are always individuals and in some cases couples and families who were willing to talk to us and reveal their fears and hopes during and after the pandemic, the routine and disruption of routine that was helping them to get through the roughly two years of the COVID-19 pandemic. This might sound like a smooth process of field work and empirical analysis, which it was not throughout. There was a period of research when we struggled to get access to Turkish everyday life beyond those representatives who almost already have a routine to talk and represent their community. In hindsight, various factors might have contributed to this issue which neither of us had encountered in our previous research. It might have been caused by the difference between the structural integration via work and other institutions on the one hand and the cultural distance that prevails between the established members of society and those who feel stigmatized through the still sub-currently operating perception of their lives as that of 'guest workers'. It certainly did not help that we made the strategic decision, influenced by the international set up of our research, to place an emphasis on English language competency, rather than 'going native' via a Turkish- or Kurdish-speaking research assistant, as done by the London team with regard to the Bangladeshi community. And finally, identifying us as researchers from a University of Applied Sciences that trains those entering the local state authority and public services might have increased the disinclination to open up the cherished privacy of a migrant family's everyday life to what might in the eyes of a potential interlocutor be seen as 'state representatives'. In sum, the lesson we learned from our research was to apply the same 'cultural sensitivity' that we later asked of those who are at the front line of public service delivery in Stuttgart.

The first of the interviews carried out in Milan was administered face to face with the head of a Peruvian association, whom the coordinator of the local unit, Marco Caselli, had met 15 years earlier during a research project (Caselli, 2009) coordinated by the ISMU Foundation (www.ismu.org) and who was one of the most prominent figures among Peruvians residing in Milan. This interview was also an opportunity to forge a link with the leader of another Peruvian association, involved in sporting activities, who was interviewed, as in the previous case, by Marco Caselli, and again face to face. The representative of a third association was then interviewed again by Marco Caselli, this time online, thanks to the suggestion of a researcher involved in various projects dedicated to Latin American communities in Italy, promoted by the ISMU Foundation.

Six interviews with Peruvian citizens without specific roles at an associative or institutional level—'non-experts'—were interviewed face to face by Alessia Rambelli, a PhD student at the Università Cattolica del Sacro Cuore in Milan. These people were selected through networks of friendship and personal acquaintances, trying to vary gender and age, and taking care to include Peruvians involved in the field of healthcare, this being a role that the representatives of the associations interviewed had reported as particularly relevant. To broaden our perspective, Silvia Malacarne then interviewed online an official of the Municipality of Milan responsible for services for immigrant citizens. Samuele Molli further conducted six interviews with leaders or active members of Catholic-inspired associations or non-Catholic Christian churches, four of them face to face and two online. Four were Peruvian citizens and two were citizens from other Latin American countries. A further face-to-face interview was conducted with the person in charge of the Archdiocese of Milan for the pastoral care of migrants. To carry out these interviews, Samuele Molli exploited the experience and some of the contacts already collected during his previous research experience conducted as part of his PhD, carried out at the Università Cattolica del Sacro Cuore and dedicated to the religious experiences of immigrant citizens.

All the interviews carried out in Milan were conducted in Italian, given the good level of knowledge of this language on the part of the interviewees. From time to time they—especially in the case of 'non-experts'—also resorted to using terms and expressions in Spanish. Most of the interviews were carried out face to face, and these interviews were the opportunity to observe the headquarters of associations and religious communities, as well as the places of life, work and meet up of the people interviewed. This allowed us to obtain useful information for our research far beyond the explicit content of the interviews themselves.

Our approach follows the general assumption that guides qualitative research, namely that people's narratives reveal (some of) the social structures and cultural frames through which their perception of fears and hopes, their conduct of routine and ambitions and their performance of identity and social functions operate. More specifically, we draw on the approach of structural hermeneutics (Alexander & Smith, 2003), which complements ethnographic 'thick description', as well as following the structural-linguistic turn in sociology by investigating 'cultural depth'. Our methodological approach can, therefore, be best described as 'sociological forensics' (Inglis, 2010), since we seek to illuminate 'the whole from the particular' by linking context-specific micro-observations to wider social structures and long-term processes of change.

1.5 Contents of the Book

The volume is organized as follows. After this introductory chapter, the first part of the book presents the particular cases addressed in the study—Turks in Stuttgart, Bangladeshis in London and Peruvians in Milan—each of which is dedicated a chapter.

The chapter dedicated to the **Bangladeshis in London** focuses on a particular borough, Tower Hamlets, which lies immediately to the east of the City of London and is widely considered to contain the heartland of the Bangladeshi community in both the metropolis and Britain, more generally. The vast majority are Muslims and since the first generation came to the area during the 1960s and 1970s, the community has become well established with a second and third generation as well as an emergent fourth generation. Although Bangladeshis in Britain are a very small minority, in Tower Hamlets they are the largest social and cultural group with a very powerful political presence and a well-established religious and community infrastructure.

After introducing the Bangladeshi community in multi-ethnic Tower Hamlets and outlining the key events during the pandemic between 2020 and 2022, the chapter draws on the interviews to address the following themes—the impact of the first 2020 lockdown, the vaccination campaign from late 2020, family dynamics, state regulations and Muslim funerals, beliefs in curse and shame, as well as the involvement of middle-class residents outside the community. The research demonstrates the important role played by Bangladeshi activists at the meso level between the macro level of the state and the micro level of people's everyday lives. Because we included in our cohort those who were not involved in community activism, our interviews with them add to our understanding of the issues that affected people 'on the ground'.

The chapter dedicated to **Turkish migrants in Stuttgart** has not the same explicit local focus as the London chapter, but nevertheless the research has focussed on hot spots of Turkish migration in Stuttgart. Feuerbach, in terms of the catchment area of its mosque, and Cannstatt, in terms of residential concentration, can be identified as such significant places. Stuttgart's history is a model of integration through the workplace or 'assembly line integration'. Many 'guest worker' families have been part and parcel of this development from the 1960s onwards and today proudly refer to themselves as 'Stuttgarters'. Meanwhile, there is a dense web of organizations with civil society and a religious affiliation that not only represents the variety of Turkish life and culture in Stuttgart, but also engages in communication and dialogue with local state institutions, thus effectively participating in the co-evolution of integration policy in Stuttgart.

The chapter initially outlines this development of integration and integration policy in Stuttgart and outlines the unfolding of the pandemic in this context. It then concentrates on analysing how the dense web of institutional and inter-personal cooperation between Turkish migrant organizations and local state bodies has helped to people to cope with the pandemic. The chapter concludes that next to obvious potentials, the pandemic has also revealed some of the limits of Stuttgart's 'integrationism'.

The following chapter, which focuses primarily on the experience of **Peruvians in Milan**, clearly reveals some significant differences compared with the previous ones. First of all, as we have already mentioned, Peruvians are predominantly Roman Catholic and, therefore, share the same religion as the Italian majority. They also speak Spanish which has the same neo-Latin origin as Italian. Secondly, Italy is a country that has been transformed from a country of emigration into a country of immigration relatively recently and Peruvians are also recent settlers. Most of those residing in Milan were born in Peru and almost all belong to the first or second generation.

The chapter shows that among Peruvians the key distinction was between regular and irregular migrants. While the experience of the pandemic for regular Peruvian citizens, who possessed official documents, was substantially similar to that recorded for Italians, the situation of undocumented Peruvians was decidedly more difficult and at times dramatically so. Furthermore, for both migrants and member of the Italian majority a particularly important role was played by civil society, since the latter frequently supported the state or compensated for the state's shortcomings, illustrating what in the chapter is identified as 'subsidiarity the other way round'.

The second part of the volume presents insights which, although starting in some cases from the specific experience of one of the contexts studied, seeks to develop some transversal reflections and analyses with respect to the three case studies around which the research project was set up in its entirety.

The chapter **Migrant Mediators as Promoters of Social Cohesion During the Pandemic: An Analysis of the Mutual Learning Process** focuses on the key role played by the so-called migrant mediators during the pandemic. These are people who are committed to promoting mutual learning processes in London, Milan and Stuttgart and are able to encourage forms of social cohesion. They generally demonstrate a strong sense of belonging to their country of origin and, at the same time, are well integrated into their country of residence. In particular, they demonstrate good familiarity in the use of both the language of the national community of reference and that of the country in which they reside. Not infrequently, they also have roles of responsibility at a social, cultural and political level in the context of reception.

After a brief insight into the impact of the health emergency on migrants and a brief description of how the concept of mutual learning can be defined with respect to the relationship between migrants and non-migrants, the value of these migrant mediators is highlighted during the crisis in the three cities, focusing on such key facilitators of mutual learning as the Covid champions in London, Peruvian migrants working on the front lines in Milanese hospitals and the German Turkish Forum in Stuttgart.

The chapter **Resisting, Reacting and Reinventing: Exploring the Role of Minority Religious Solidarities in Milan and London During the Pandemic** examines the role of religious institutions, such as churches and mosques, during and after the pandemic. Their ways of resisting and reacting to the emergency are explored as well as the ways in which they adapted their religious beliefs and practices when institutional measures, such as lockdown and social distancing, were imposed from above. Analytically, the chapter adopts a city-level perspective with the aim of exploring the concrete impact of macro processes on the lives of migrant minorities. It discusses the specific cases of Latin American Catholics and Pentecostals, especially those of Peruvian origin, in Milan and Bangladeshi

Muslims in London, and considers how their settlement was shaped by different ways in which religious diversity was regulated.

The evidence collected through our research project is assembled under various themes such as (a) the minorities' religious welfare efforts which sought to tackle people's socio-economic needs and embodied a sense of mission for the needy, (b) the civic role played by religious welfarism in engaging with lockdown restrictions and reinforcing or restricting compliance and/or adherence with public institutions, and (c) the impact of the emergency on religious beliefs and practices. The chapter sheds light on why and how religions played a crucial role for minority populations at a time of profound change dictated by a global health crisis. It also provides a glimpse of the future by identifying the 'signs of the times' in the aftermath of the pandemic.

The chapter **The Importance of Urban Culture as a Middle Ground Between State and Ethnic Minorities in Negotiating (Im)mobilities: The London Context** considers the complexities of class, gender, cultural dynamics and cultural change within an urban context, as well as the positions people occupy or come to occupy. The primary focus here is the London context, with special reference to the Bangladeshi population of Tower Hamlets during the COVID-19 pandemic. The chapter also explores issues around technological spaces, communication and digital spaces and freedoms as well as the impact of belonging to local social networks (rather than to, say, communities), issues around elasticity in social systems and overarching structural systems (the macro, meso and micro) that partly shape our interactions with institutions.

The chapter **Good (Local) Governance and State Capacity: Continuity and Difference in Times of Pandemic and Beyond** analyses some key elements emerging from the whole research process. It turns towards an investigation of 'good governance' in times of pandemic and beyond. It starts by locating the chapter within debates concerning 'rescaling' and 'multi-level governance' and highlights the analytical importance of local-level policy for both ad hoc pandemic emergency governance and long-term integration governance. In terms of 'sociological forensics' it draws on interview material to uncover the pattern of cooperation and conflict between migrant minorities and local government institutions in each of the three city locales. Attention shifts from conventional 'public administration' in Stuttgart to the ambivalent role played by the NHS as an 'anchor institution' in London and then to the role played by the Roman Catholic Church in Milan as a substitute public service provider.

The chapter concludes by suggesting that there might be a turn towards 'humble governance' in all three city locales.

Finally, the **Conclusion: Towards a Sociological Understanding of Layered Resilience** supports our initial claim that the interplay between 'state capacity' and the 'capacity to aspire' finds its Archimedean Point in the fuzzy field of 'layered resilience'. The basic insights emerging from our research provide substance to this claim and are sketched out in the concluding chapter. The conclusion also provides suggestions for future research within the matrix of migrant population/local state/ pandemic/integration. After outlining some insights from our research in London, Stuttgart and Milan, that might contribute to a sociological understanding of the concept of 'layered resilience', the chapter concludes with a brief view about continuity and difference between COVID-19 and previous pandemics that shaped world history.

References

Alexander, J., & Smith, P. (2003). The Strong Program in Cultural Sociology: Elements of a Structural Hermeneutics. In J. Alexander (Ed.), *The Meanings of Social Life* (pp. 11–26). Oxford University Press.

Appadurai, A. (2013). *The Future as Cultural Fact: Essays on the Global Condition*. Verso.

Apuzzo, M., & Kirkpatrick, D. D. (2020, April 1) Covid-19 Changed How the World Does Science Together. *The New York Times*.

Bauböck, R., & Orgad, L., (Eds). (2020). Cities vs. States: Should Urban Citizenship be Emancipated from Nationality? *EUI (European Univ. Institute) Working Paper RSCAS*, 2020/16.

Beck, U. (1992). *Risk Society: Towards a New Modernity*. Sage.

Bermudez, J. M., & Mancini, J. A. (2013). Families Fuertes: Family Resilience Among Latinos. In D. S. Becvar (Ed.), *Handbook of Family Resilience* (pp. 215–227). Springer.

Black, K., & Lobo, M. (2008). A Conceptual Review of Family Resilience Factors. *Journal of Family Nursing, 14*(1), 33–55.

Bourbeau, P. (2015). Migration, Resilience and Security: Responses to New Inflows of Asylum Seekers and Migrants. *Journal of Ethnic and Migration Studies, 41*(12), 1958–1977.

Campomori, F., & Caponio, T. (2017). Immigrant Integration Policymaking in Italy: Regional Policies in a Multi-level Governance Perspective. *International Review of Administrative Sciences, 83*(2), 303–321. https://doi.org/10.1177/ 0020852315611238

Caselli, M. (2009). *Vite transnazionali? Peruviani e peruviane a Milano.* FrancoAngeli.

Clement, J., Esposito, G., & Crutzen, N. (2023). Municipal Pathways in Response to COVID-19: A Strategic Management Perspective on Local Public Administration Resilience. *Administration & Society, 55*(1), 3–29.

Davvetas, V., Ulqinaku, A., & Abi, G. S. (2022). Local Impact of Global Crises, Institutional Trust, and Consumer Well-Being: Evidence from the COVID-19 Pandemic. *Journal of International Marketing, 30*(2), 73–101.

Doty, J. (2016). Resilience in Immigrant and Refugee Families. In J. Ballard, E. Wieling, C. Solheim, & L. Dwanyen (Eds.), *Immigrant and Refugee Families: Global Perspectives on Displacement and Resettlement Experiences* (pp. 176–197). University of Minnesota Library Publishing.

Drinkwater, S., Eade, J., & Garapich, M. (2008). Britain's Ethnic Diversity and Recent Migration from the A8 Countries. In A. Krasteva (Ed.), *Immigration and Integration: European Experiences* (pp. 40–54). Sofia.

Eade, J. (1989). *The Politics of Community.* Avebury.

Eade, J. (Ed.). (1997a). *Living the Global City: Globalization as Local Process.* Routledge.

Eade, J. (1997b). Nationalism, Community and the Islamization of Space in London. In B. D. Metcalf (Ed.), *Making Muslim Space in North America and Europe* (pp. 217–233). University of California Press.

Eade, J. (2007). Economic Migrants or Hyphenated British? Writing about Difference in London's East End. In S. Gupta & T. Omoniyi (Eds.), *The New Orders of Difference: Cultural Discourses and Texts of Economic Migration in Europe, Asia, and Africa* (pp. 27–36). Ashgate.

Eade, J. (2013). Bengalis in Britain: Migration, State Controls and Settlement. In J. Chatterj & D. Washbrook (Eds.), *Routledge Handbook of the South Asian Diaspora* (pp. 280–294). Routledge.

Eade, J., & Garapich, M. (2009a). Settling or Surviving in London: The Experience of Poles and Other 'A8' Migrants in a Global City Borough. In J. Eade & Y. Valkanova (Eds.), *Accession and Migration: Changing Policy, Society, and Culture in an Enlarged Europe* (pp. 143–166). Ashgate.

Eade, J., & Garapich, M. (2009b). Roots and Routes: Permanent Settlement and Circular Migration in the EU. In G. Koch & A. Franke (Eds.), *Kulturelle Vielfalt als Gestaltungsaufgabe. Ethnologische Beiträge aus diversen Praxisfeldern* (pp. 33–45). Röhrig Verlag.

Elliott, A., & Turner, B. S. (2012). *On Society.* Polity.

Emilsson, H. (2015). A National Turn of Local Integration Policy: Multi-Level Governance Dynamics in Denmark and Sweden. *Comparative Migration Studies, 3*(7), 1–16. https://doi.org/10.1186/s40878-015-0008-5

Fukuyama, F. (2020, March 30). The Thing that Determines a Country' Resistance to the Coronavirus. *The Atlantic.*

Furceri, D., Loungani, P., Ostry, J. D., & Pizzuto, P. (2022). Will COVID-19 Have Long-Lasting Effects on Inequality? Evidence from Past Pandemics. *The Journal of Economic Inequality, 20*, 811–839.

Galandini, S., Mulvey, G., & Lessard-Phillips, L. (2019). Stuck between Mainstreaming and Localism: Views on the Practice of Migrant Integration in a Devolved Policy Framework. *Journal of International Migration and Integration, 20*, 685–702. https://doi.org/10.1007/s12134-018-0626-5

Garcés-Mascareñas, B., & Penninx, R. (Eds.). (2016). *Integration Processes and Policies in Europe*. Springer.

Gielis, R. (2011). The Value of Single-Site Ethnography in the Global Era: Studying Transnational Experiences in the Migrant House. *Area, 43*(3), 257–263.

Glick Schiller, N., & Çağlar, A. (Eds.). (2011). *Locating Migration: Rescaling Cities and Migrants*. Cornell University Press.

Green, S. (2007). Divergent Traditions, Converging Responses: Immigration and Integration Policy in the UK and Germany. *German Politics, 16*(1), 95–115.

Hepburn, E., & Zapata-Barrero, R. (2014). Introduction: Immigration Policies in Multilevel States. In E. Hepburn & R. Zapata-Barrero (Eds.), *The Politics of Immigration in Multilevel States: Governance and Political Parties* (pp. 3–18). Palgrave.

Hidalgo, D. M., Nunn, P. D., & Beazley, H. (2021). Uncovering Multilayered Vulnerability and Resilience in Rural Villages in the Pacific: A Case Study of Ono Island, Fiji. *Ecology and Society, 26*(1), 26.

Holley, P. (2020). Being Cosmopolitan and Anti-Cosmopolitan—The Covid-19 Pandemic as a Cosmopolitan Moment. *The European Sociologist, 45*.

Holsten, J., & Appadurai, A. (1996). Cities and Citizenship. *Public Culture, 8*, 187–204.

Inglis, T. (2010). Sociological Forensics: Illuminating the Whole from the Particular. *Sociology, 44*(3), 507–522.

Johnson, D. R., Scheitle, C. P., & Ecklund, E. H. (2021). Beyond the In-Person Interview? How Interview Quality Varies Across In-person, Telephone, and Skype Interviews. *Social Science Computer Review, 39*(6), 1142–1158. https://doi.org/10.1177/0894439319893612

Joppke, C. (2004). Ethnic Diversity and the State. *British Journal of Sociology, 55*(3), 451–463.

Link, B. G. (2008). Epidemological Sociology and the Social Shaping of Population Health. *Journal of Health and Social Behaviour, 49*, 367–384.

Lucassen, L. (2004, February 27–28). *Old Wine in New Bottles? Turks and Poles in Germany and the Importance of Historical Comparisons*. Workshop on the Integration of Immigrants from Turkey in Austria, Germany and Holland: Bogazici University, Istanbul.

Maurović, I., Liebenberg, L., & Ferić, M. (2020). A Review of Family Resilience: Understanding the Concept and Operationalization Challenges to Inform Research and Practice. *Child Care in Practice, 26*(4), 337–357.

McGhee, D., Moreh, C., & Vlachantoni, A. (2017). An 'Undeliberate Determinacy'? The Changing Migration Strategies of Polish Migrants in the UK in Times of Brexit. *Journal of Ethnic and Migration Studies, 43*(13), 2109–2130.

Mu, G. M. (2021). Sociologising Resilience through Bourdieu's Field Analysis: Misconceptualisation, Conceptualisation, and Reconceptualisation. *British Journal of Sociology of Education, 42*(1), 15–31. https://doi.org/10.1080/01425692.2020.1847634

Obrist, B., Pfeiffer, C., & Henley, R. (2010). Multi-Layered Social Resilience: A New Approach in Mitigation Research. *Progress in Development Studies, 10*(4), 283–293.

OECD. (2020). *What Is the Impact of the COVID-19 Pandemic on Immigrants and Their Children?* [oecd.org/coronavirus]

Ogueji, I. A., Okoloba, M. M., & Demoko Ceccaldi, B. M. (2022). Coping Strategies of Individuals in the United Kingdom during the COVID-19 Pandemic. *Current Psychology, 41*(11), 7493–7499.

Penninx, R., & Garcés-Mascareñas, B. (2016). The Concept of Integration as an Analytical Tool and as a Policy Concept. In R. Penninx & B. Garcés-Mascareñas (Eds.), *Integration Processes and Policies in Europe*. Springer.

Penninx, R., Kraal, K., Martiniello, M., & Vertovec, S. (2020/2004). *Citizenship in European Cities: Immigrants, Local Politics and Integration Policies.* Routledge.

Rivera, C. P., Quesada, J., & Holmes, S. M. (2019). Structural Vulnerability and New Perspectives in Social Medicine on the Health of Immigrants: Interview with James Quesada and Seth M. Holmes. *Salud Colectiva*, 12.

Rodríguez-Caballero, C. V., & Vera-Valdés, J. E. (2020). Long-Lasting Economic Effects of Pandemics: Evidence on Growth and Unemployment. *Econometrics, 8*(3), 37.

Schönwälder, K. (2020). Diversity and Political Practice. *Ethnic and Racial Studies, 43*(11), 1929–1941.

Triandafyllidou, A. (2020). Spaces of Solidarity and Spaces of Exception at the Times of Covid-19. *International MIgration, 58*(3), 261–263.

Vertovec, S. (2020). Global Migration and the 'Great Reshaping'. *Max Planck Research, 3*, 20–25.

PART I

Three Case Studies: London, Stuttgart, and Milan

CHAPTER 2

Bangladeshis in London and Tower Hamlets: Community Activism and the Local State

John Eade

2.1 Introducing the London Borough of Tower Hamlets and Its Bangladeshi Population

According to the 2021 Census of England and Wales, 644,881 people identified themselves as Bangladeshis or 1.1 per cent of the total population. This represented a 42.9 per cent increase from the 451,529 recorded in the 2011 census[1]—a massive increase that largely reflected the youthful demographic of Bangladeshi settlement. The vast majority of Bangladeshis lived in English urban areas and almost half (322,054) were located across the Greater London area.[2] The most popular London borough for

[1] https://www.ons.gov.uk/peoplepopulationandcommunity/culturalidentity/ethnicity/bulletins/ethnicgroupenglandandwales/census2021.xssx, accessed 5/4/2023.

[2] https://www.google.com/search?q=bangladeshi+population+london+2022&oq=Bangladeshi+population+London+2&aqs=chrome.1.69i57j33i160l5j33i21l2j33i22i29i30l2.26335j0j4&sourceid=chrome&ie=UTF-8, accessed 5/4/2023.

J. Eade (✉)
University of Roehampton, London, UK
e-mail: J.Eade@roehampton.ac.uk

M. Caselli et al. (eds.), *Migrants' (Im)mobilities in Three European Urban Contexts*, Europe in a Global Context,
https://doi.org/10.1007/978-3-031-53773-8_2

Bangladeshis was Tower Hamlets, which bordered London's global financial hub and historic centre—the City of London. By 2021, 312,273 people were recorded as living in the borough, of which 107,333 or 34.6 per cent were Bangladeshis, i.e. by far the largest ethnic group.[3] Although Tower Hamlets was widely considered to be heart of the Bangladeshi community, the neighbouring boroughs of Newham and Waltham Forest to the east and Camden Town to the north also contained substantial numbers of Bangladeshis.

Despite the dominant presence of Bangladeshis in Tower Hamlets, the borough had attracted other minority ethnic groups. As the borough profile noted:

> The borough is ranked as the 16th most ethnically diverse local authority in England in terms of the mix of different ethnic group populations. More than two thirds of our residents belong to minority ethnic groups. ... the most significant population growth in recent years was among EU nationals.[4]

Although ethnicity was socially and culturally important, the ties of social class cut across ethnic boundaries, reflecting the long history of the area as a predominantly working class area (Eade, 1989, 2000; Glynn, 2016). The southern wards clustered around a number of docks, which were built during the late eighteenth and early nineteenth century and which extended along the north side of the River Thames into the neighbouring borough of Newham and across the river into Bermondsey. The northern wards largely hosted small factories, breweries and retail and wholesale businesses and this is where the first generation of Bangladeshi settlers, who arrived during the 1960s and 1970s, settled in large numbers, working in the local garment factories, restaurants and cafes, small shops and manual jobs (Carey & Shukur, 1985; Eade, 1989, 2000).

Brick Lane, near the borough's western border with the City of London, became internationally famous for its ethnic mix of restaurants, cafes and shops. Its mosque (see Fig. 2.1) represented the long history of migration to the area, since it was built by French Huguenot refugees in the 1740s as a Protestant chapel, was used by East European Jewish settlers as a synagogue from the late nineteenth century and became a mosque during the

[3] https://www.towerhamlets.gov.uk/News_events/2022/December-2022/New-Tower-Hamlets-census-data-released.aspx

[4] https://www.towerhamlets.gov.uk/Documents/Borough_statistics/Research-briefings/Population_2_BP2018.pdf

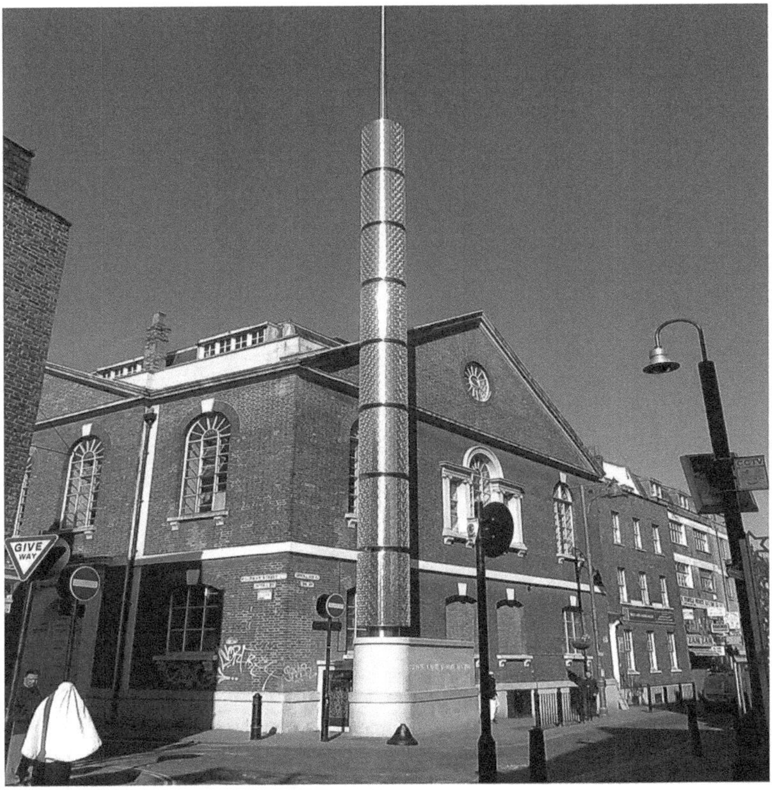

Fig. 2.1 Brick Lane Mosque (photograph by the author)

1970s (Alexander, 2011; Eade, 1989, 2000). A short walk southwards on the busy thoroughfare of Whitechapel Road was another well-known religious landmark—the purpose-built East London Mosque (see Fig. 2.2) which opened its doors in 1986 and now provided a range of facilities, such as shops, housing, an Islamic school and a funeral service (for a history of the East London Mosque, see Ansari, 2011, 2013; Carey & Shukur, 1985).

During the 1980s and 1990s many members of the first generation settled down rather than return to Bangladesh—a process that was encouraged by the arrival of wives and dependants and the increasingly restrictive nature of immigration controls. Since the late 1990s the gradual

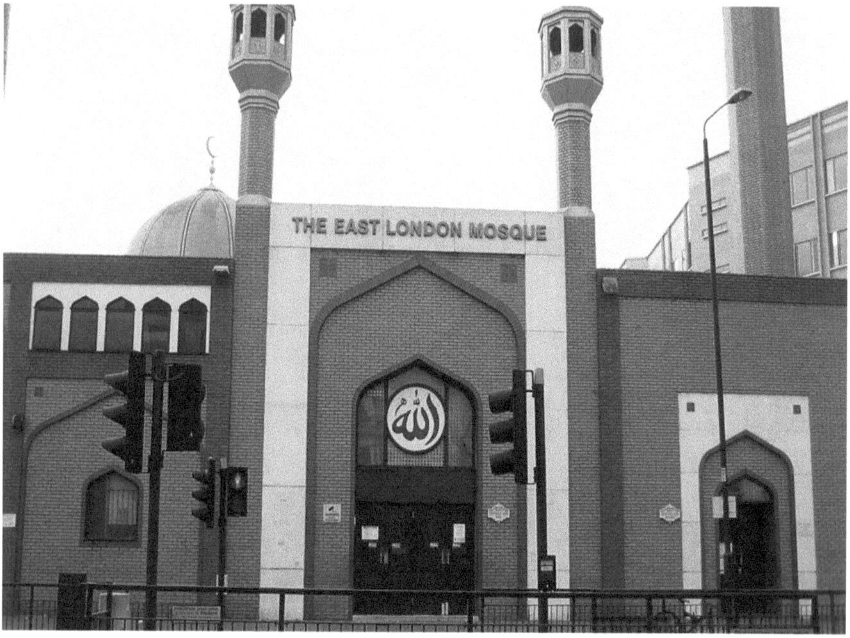

Fig. 2.2 East London Mosque (photograph by the author)

disappearance of the local garment factories has increased the reliance of the second and the third generation on employment in restaurants, cafes and shops as well as taxi driving, food delivery and more middle-class jobs in local offices, schools, health and welfare provision, local government and other areas of the service sector. Some members of the third generation, especially those who attended university and acquired professional qualifications, were also able to find white-collar jobs in the nearby City of London and the 'Docklands' area to the south of the borough. Docklands had developed from the 1980s around the redundant docks and its towering offices and expensive residential blocks radically changed the local landscape and the social character of what had been a predominantly working class area (Butler, 2007; Brownhill, 2010). The Bangladeshi population has become more economically and socially diverse, therefore, as a social and economic divide developed between white-collar workers and those confined to insecure, unskilled or semi-skilled occupations. As noted in the borough profile cited above, Tower Hamlets was the second most deprived London borough in 2017 'with high rates of poverty, child poverty, unemployment and pay inequality' and the divisions within the Bangladeshi population reflected this deprivation.

2.2 The Pandemic in UK: A Timeline and Its Differential Impact

The first cases were reported at the end of January 2020 but the government delayed introducing a national lockdown until March 23. Like many other European countries, the government eventually ended the lockdown but sought to restrict social interaction by limiting the number of people could meet socially and keeping leisure venues such as cafes, restaurants and pubs closed as well as introducing on May 28 a 'test and trace' system to prevent COVID infections spreading. In autumn the rising numbers of infections led to a second lockdown for five weeks from November 5. The invention of vaccines by private pharmaceutical companies enabled the government through the National Health System (NHS) to begin a vaccination programme from December 8, 2020, but imposed a third lockdown after the Christmas and New Year festivities on January 4, 2021. Towards the end of March 2021 half the UK population had been vaccinated and the declining number of infections led the government to relax restrictions on public meetings during July 2021. The remaining legal obstacles to mixing were ended in February 2022.[5]

When the pandemic struck, there was widespread concern about the differential impact on the UK population (Platt & Warwick, 2020). Since many Bangladeshis were employed in the public sector, they were unable to self-isolate through home working and their accommodation was often overcrowded and lacked access to outside space. Social and cultural norms discouraged social distancing, while there were problems of communicating information from the central and local government and local NHS institutions such as hospitals and health centres. Critics of the government and NHS also argued that minorities, in general, had long been subjected to 'institutional racism.'

Health provision is administered by the local authorities, i.e. the borough councils. Although borough councils lost control of housing as a major resource during the 1980s, it is still useful to distinguish between

[5] Hugh Pym, 'Covid: Farewell Downing St briefings (for now, at least)', https://www.bbc.com/news/health-60510852, 27/2/2022, accessed 6/3/2022.

local and central government in terms of local and central state institutions. The National Health Service is closely linked to the state, and during 2020 and 2021, the weekly televised presentations of government policy, two NHS representatives stood either side of a government minister to demonstrate this intimate, albeit tense relationship.

During the first wave of the pandemic (March to May 2020) Bangladeshi elders appeared to be particularly affected. As conditions eased during the summer and autumn of 2020 before the second lockdown, there was anecdotal evidence that local and central state messages about observing state regulations and later taking up the new vaccine, reinforced by the NHS, had a significant impact on social mixing and vaccination rates.

2.3 Impact of COVID-19 on Bangladeshis in Tower Hamlets and Their Response

Regular updates were issued on the pandemic's impact on the UK population, and it appeared that by March 2021 vaccination rates in Tower Hamlets were some of the lowest not only in London but in the UK:

> NHS Tower Hamlets Clinical Commissioning Group (CCG) has one of the lowest vaccination rates for over 60s in London, according to the latest NHS data. Between 8th December 2020 and 7th March 2021, 66.3% of over 60s in the area had been given their first dose. Local London Assembly Member Unmesh Desai AM has praised the local efforts behind the vaccine rollout so far, but has warned that Tower Hamlets could be "left behind" if factors such as vaccine supply and hesitancy were not robustly addressed. He said that it "isn't about a race against other parts of the capital or the country, but a race against the virus". … NHS data shows that ten of the worst performing Parliamentary constituencies in the country are all in London.[6]

Many groups and individuals were involved in encouraging local residents to observe state regulations and engage with the vaccination programme, but in the case of Bangladeshi residents the role played by community and political activists was not only important but was highly informative about the relationship between the state and citizens more generally. In other words, between the macro level of central and local state capacity and NHS provision, on the one hand, and the micro level of

[6] https://www.london.gov.uk/press-releases/assembly/unmesh-desai/tower-hamlets-ccg-has-low-vaccination-rate accessed June 6, 2021.

everyday life, there was a meso level occupied by a range of local Bangladeshi activists among others. These activists operated through both local and transnational networks since Bangladeshis in London and other parts of the UK were closely linked to relatives in Bangladesh and knew about the impact of COVID in Bangladesh and other countries in S. Asia.

The central state and the NHS tried to pursue a universalist response to the challenges presented by the pandemic. Lockdown restrictions and the vaccination programme were officially introduced without regard to differences of class, gender, ethnicity or race. However, from March 2020 critics pointed to the ways in which the universalist aims of the state were constrained by these differences. At the level of the local state, however, this universalist strategy was implemented through policies and practices which took particular social and cultural forces into consideration. Hence, the significance of the political and community networks in helping Bangladeshi residents to adapt to the health crisis.

Care must be taken to avoid viewing Bangladeshis as a homogenous group. Intersectional analysis has demonstrated the ways in which people's everyday lives were shaped by the complex intersection of gender, sexuality, generation, language, religion and occupation. Bangladeshis were intimately involved in this intersectional complexity so that some fared better during the pandemic than others. Well-educated Bangladeshis, who lived in spacious accommodation and were able to work from home, enjoyed similar life chances to white professionals, for example, and experienced the pandemic differently from other Bangladeshis, who were far less fortunate.

The ten activists, whom we contacted, were similar in many respects to these well-educated Bangladeshis but their effectiveness as activists revealed the importance of social networks that had been developed since the 1980s between political and community groups which had led to Bangladeshis constituting the majority of borough councillors and, thereby, gaining access to the control of scarce public resources such as jobs and amenities. These networks also included those who represented the housing cooperatives that took over control of accommodation previously administered by the borough council. Although most activists were male, the two female activists we interviewed were part of the Bangladeshi female cohort that had also entered local political and community arenas—both members of parliament for Tower Hamlets were Bangladeshi women, for example. The five 'non-experts' were involved in different networks, since they did not engage with the political and community group activism which had developed since the 1980s.

2.4 The Impact of the First 2020 Lockdown

Because the state institutions including the NHS were ill prepared for the onslaught of the COVID-19 virus in early 2020, the imposition of the first lockdown in late March caused a massive disruption of health provision and people's everyday lives.

Our interlocutors usually focused on the local or national level but Arun Chowdhury,[7] who was a Bangladeshi Hindu working as a legal adviser and administrator for a prominent Bangladeshi community organization, placed the emotional impact of the pandemic on health professionals in a more global context:

> *Government is not prepared for this unprecedented situation… even doctors …I got at least 20 close friends, they are doctors [in Bangladesh] …[and] one … at Nova Scotia [Canada] he called me and said: 'I do not know what to do' because they never experienced this before … Even doctors cannot touch the patients … One of my friends lives in North London said … 'I cannot sleep at night' … and he burst into tears … 'I am literally doing nothing for them… I am afraid to touch her or him' … That was a crucial and heartbreaking time.*
>
> *The whole machine was broken, because they were actually not ready … to the experience of this scenario … They were panicking.*

During this time many went to hospital and never survived. As one of our activists poignantly declared:

> *I am so sad and I am so angry against this Corona because I lost one of my friend's sons because of this Corona… He was only 34 years old … He had asthma as well … He had gone to hospital with his grandma but his grandma came back and he didn't … which is very, very sad.*

However, Afia Begum, who was a funeral director, provided a much more positive account of what happened during the early stages of the pandemic in 2020. She was very impressed and surprised by how Bangladeshi families, hospital staff and officials in the coroners' office collaborated at the local level:

> *I'm talking about the first lockdown … and I'm looking back to it, what really, really amazed me is that how amazing the families were that were bereaved … I'm not talking just about the families, I'm talking about the coroners, the*

[7] In the interests of anonymity we have given our interlocutors fictional names.

hospitals, the pandemic just made everyone become very collaborative ... What I found was that people were just so, so helpful ... I would have registrars ringing me up in the early hours and saying we haven't got the paperwork ... It's unheard of, it's unprecedented what people were doing ... just to be able to keep the services going ... making sure people were getting the funeral their loved ones wanted ... So there were issues for sure, but if I felt there was a lot of cooperation.

Certain areas of local health care, therefore, such as the one where Afia operated, avoided what appeared to be initial confusion and a lack of preparedness where many people contracted the virus and tragically died in hospital and care homes without the support of family and friends. During 2020 coordination between state institutions gradually improved and the engagement with local residents strengthened with the support of community activists. As Irfan Iqbal, a borough councillor, explained during his interview which took place on December 1, 2021, when the vaccination programme was in full swing during 2021:

Our public health team is in constant liaison with the hospitals ... with the care places as well because there was a big breakout in care homes and we're much more aware of what's happening or keeping tabs on what's happening in local hospitals and there's constant communication with the doctors and hospital teams and we also have local Covid Champions, who were building people up to spread the message ... They meet every once a week and discuss what the next steps are and what can be done to do different things. And, obviously, the whole Covid discussion went from isolation to staying away to the vaccine and now to the second jab and then to the booster ... and it's how you try and get more people through ...Those initiatives have worked.

2.5 Volunteering: The Covid Champions, Community Centres and Political Activists

The Covid Champions scheme was funded by the borough council and began at the beginning of the pandemic in 2020 when around '2,300 people signed up as volunteers.'[8] Their remit was 'to help neighbours and others who were socially isolated, including those advised to self-isolate'

[8] https://www.eastlondonadvertiser.co.uk/news/local-council/20955424.covid-community-champions-get-tower-hamlets-council-cash-carry-helping-neighbours/, accessed 5/7/2023.

by, for example, 'transporting protective equipment to carers' homes, delivering shopping to the housebound, helping in community kitchens and distributing food supplies to voluntary organisations and local food banks.'[9]

After the interview with Irfan Iqbal we decided to include a Covid Champion in our cohort of ten 'experts' and Shamea Mia arranged a meeting with Abdus Saleh in a Bangladeshi cafe on Brick Lane on December 3, 2022. He explained that he and the other volunteers drew on their extensive local networks: 'Our work is to make connections with each other ... We have good connections with lots of people ... and I have good connections with media. Wherever people are needed, we make connections.' The volunteers helped in a variety of ways:

> *Different people did different things ... For example, if you couldn't take money out of the bank ... a lot of the time, we did bank transfers for people... There were about 50, 60 of us Covid Champions working together ... There are about 50,000 people living here ... so we couldn't help everyone.*

He then described how he helped a family, which had migrated from Italy, when one of their members had died during the pandemic:

> *Someone died, who came from Italy, from Green Street and didn't have any family here and didn't have any money ... To bury someone here costs around £4000 ... It's not an easy amount especially for someone who has just come over ... So they got in touch with me, they phoned me and we all went over to help ... So we helped out as much as we could altogether, we were all involved ... We collected money for the deceased, someone gave £10, someone gave £20 ... But it's not my credit ... we all worked together ... Someone even gave £200 ... We all donated.*

He and his fellow Bangladeshi Muslim volunteers, in particular, liaised with the local families, doctors, hospitals and the mosques:

> *People, who passed away from Covid, their families couldn't go but we went to help out ... We liaised with the doctors, the hospitals ... And you have to wait two, three, four weeks for a body ... So we liaised and ... then only five people were allowed at the funeral at the Janazah [mosque] prayer—five to ten people maximum ... the highest number was 25.*

[9] https://www.eastlondonadvertiser.co.uk/news/local-council/20955424.covid-community-champions-get-tower-hamlets-council-cash-carry-helping-neighbours/, accessed 5/7/2023.

The Covid Champions also helped with delivering food to people who were obliged to stay at home and had not subscribed to the home delivery service provided by supermarkets chains such as Tesco and Sainsbury. However, others were involved in supporting local residents during the height of the pandemic in 2020 and 2021. Free food was handed out at food banks run by local community centres. During a walk around the Spitalfields area in late April 2020 when restrictions on movement began to ease towards the end of the first lockdown, we encountered a long queue of Bangladeshi women waiting to collect food parcels at the Osmani Centre, a large community centre which, according to its website, 'offers a range of highly versatile and creative spaces from Community Hall, Training Room to a Youth Club facilities and an Active Studio. Osmani Centre is a great place for conferences, seminars, meetings, training days, wedding reception or cultural functions.'[10] Vans were delivering food to two other centres in close proximity—Spitalfields' Roman Catholic church and a disused shop which served as a distribution centre run by a charity based in north London. As Abdus Saleh, the Covid Champion, noted local political activists were also involved:

> *The local councillors … they did their bit in terms of putting out literature in Bengali and I'm aware of some of the councillors … working in their own neighbourhoods in terms of supporting people who lived isolation, single people … elderly people … Many councillors I'm aware of dropping food off to vulnerable adults who were living on their own … I'm also aware of councillors running food banks … so many councillors … Definitely, Spitalfields councillors were involved in distributing food and being involved with food banks.*

Personal relationships between community and political activists played a crucial role in mobilising and communicating across the borough during the lockdown as Nazir Shah explained:

> *Because I'm a community worker and I know the councillor personally … I could email them or I could phone them and they would respond straight away … Now for an ordinary person, I don't know how easy or difficult it might have been during the lockdown … I really don't know to be honest, you'd have to ask a local person … But for me, it wasn't a problem … because of my community involvement and because I live locally and I know some of the councillors and I've known them for years … It's that relationships that probably enables me to have easy access to them.*

[10] https://www.osmanicentre.org/about-us/, accessed 22/9/2023.

Yet, although the work of Covid Champions like Abdus Saleh and other activists like those whom we contacted was very important, the general impact of losing relatives and friends may well have had even greater significance in encouraging people to take the pandemic seriously and comply with official regulations. As Nazir Shah noted, the second wave which took place during late 2020 and early 2021 forced people to be more compliant with state regulations:

> *I think during the first lockdown … many within the community were not aware of the seriousness of the illness because it's something that was unknown to all of us. And because we hadn't seen anyone with Corona and we hadn't seen the symptoms or how one would suffer … I don't think people took it seriously. The second wave … I think hit home harder … especially with the Bengali community because I think in the second round, we lost a lot of people in the community … Lots of people were not only hospitalised but they also died … I think by then people became much more fearful of the illness and perhaps took some of the preventative measures more seriously.*

2.6 Vaccination Campaign from Late 2020: Encouraging Bangladeshi Engagement

The invention of vaccines—initially by the pharmaceutical firm, Astra Zeneca and then by Pfizer and Moderna—was hailed by the government as a breakthrough and the local network of health authorities and health centres was deployed to support the vaccination programme from December 2020 with the elderly as a priority. There was a degree of scepticism about the official advice transmitted by the central government but scientists, NHS officials and minority representatives helped to promote greater trust and acceptance. As noted by the young Bangladeshi Muslim doctor we interviewed:

> *What I could see was the majority of the people were encouraging others to take the advice because the advice wasn't only coming from the government—it was coming from scientists and the NHS experts.*
>
> *And you had prominent Black people, minority race people and people from religious institutions encouraging people, so that played an important role in the uptake in the end, even though there was quite a bit of scepticism at the beginning.*

According to this doctor, the scepticism was encouraged by confusing messages as well as businesses profiting from the emergency:

> *People trust scientists ... but sometimes there are disagreements between scientists and that helped generate more scepticism. There is also scepticism from companies making money out of the pandemic ... the vaccine companies and companies like Amazon ... they made a lot of money because people did a lot of shopping online and bought a lot of stuff.*

Irfan Iqbal, the borough councillor representing the Labour Party, not surprisingly perhaps, emphasised the part played by the Labour-controlled council in encouraging Bangladeshi Muslims to be vaccinated and liaising closely with a variety of people such as doctors, those running the East London Mosque, journalists and social influencers:

> *When the pandemic started on the vaccine stuff ... we had a huge campaign around those ... sort of hesitance from people to take the vaccine. People were ... saying: 'There's ... vaccines made out of sort of pork, and animal stuff, and gelatine.' All that stuff ... So that we had a big campaign with local doctors, Bangladeshi doctors, Muslim doctors saying: 'Actually, this isn't the case, take the vaccine.' And so on ... One of the things we did as a council is we rolled out the vaccine to East London Mosque ... for people to get vaccinated ... and that helped ... We were giving out all sorts of vaccine papers and we were putting out into Bangladeshi media channels. We were telling people to come together and ... listen to what was happening or what was being said ... We're sort of looking at how to get young influencers, on social media to spread the message as well.*

Irfan also raised the issue of the relationship between the generations:

> *It's the younger generation, and a lot of them influencing the parents saying: 'This isn't actually true ... Don't take the vaccine'... And we had that sort of big, big argument in the community going on.*

Although considerable effort was put into informing people about the advantages of vaccination and countering 'fake news,' reliance on information technology raised the issue of digital exclusion. As Irfan again explained:

> *Digitally, we tried to engage a lot of young people, especially younger ages in school, so but then you actually figure out that there's a whole other sort of dimension of digital exclusion happening here as well... so the family's on the poverty line and so on ... I'm not doing well financially, if there are two or three kids and they probably had one device ... and a lot of the time it was their*

mum's or dad's mobile phone, or probably one device and they have to share it between two or three people so that the exclusion was really quite real.

As we have already seen, some Bangladeshis living in the borough were recent migrants and some were undocumented, resulting in another form of exclusion. As Nazir Shah, for example, noted:

There is a large migrant community, as you put it ... Bangladeshi migrants who have recently come from Bangladesh or even from Europe ... Bangladesh students and some other ... I think from the UK ... [who] have gone to other European countries and have re-entered the UK ... and they weren't registered as such ... and they were working mainly in ... Bengali shops and other businesses ... and during the lockdown the majority of the couriers... or the Vespa drivers are all of Bengali origin and most of them are not local ... established ... I think they are recent arrivals from Bangladesh.

These recent Bangladeshis migrants, especially those who were undocumented, found it very difficult to access local resources according to Nazir Shah:

They ... weren't able to access the support that was provided, say, ... by the council or the NHS ... because within the migrant community many ... aren't legally here and because of this they were fearful in that how would they go about for help ... And I'm aware that [some groups were] advocating for vaccinations for those who aren't registered here or don't have legal status and I think there was a campaign to get those people vaccinated ... because they're not legal. They didn't have GPs and probably couldn't go to clinics.

2.7 Economic Considerations

Those, who were unable to work from home, were at high risk of contracting the virus. The economic consequences of contracting the virus were vividly described by one of the Bangladeshi homemakers who had migrated from Italy:

At that time, we had a horrible time ... everyone was fearful ... If schools were open, one felt bad; if your husband had to go to work, one felt bad ... What if he brought the virus home from work? We couldn't see anybody... we could only go shopping and even that had rules we had to follow like keeping distances etc ... That was a very bad experience

If he doesn't go to work … the benefits that we receive are not substantial to run the family … We have the extra expenditure; where would that come from? … How could he have gone to work during the pandemic? So at that time, we had to suffer.

[Interviewer]: What does your husband do?

My husband is a taxi driver so he was at home during that time … He has to give rent for the taxi and then he has to pay for the car insurance… and there are a lot of things to pay for the car here and if he doesn't work, where will that money come from?

Abdus Sobhan also had to go out to work. He was a journalist, who was employed by a local Bengali language television and radio station, and he explained that when the first lockdown ended and it was possible to meet people his manager explained that:

Those, who read the news, would need to be helped or if there was a patient further away who was a bit ill, we would have to go to them … and I couldn't say no, there was no alternative … No one had the courage.

After interviewing people who had a mild attack of the virus, he would return to his office where he met with an apprehensive reception: 'Whenever I went into the office, everyone used to tell me that I would bring the disease into the office with me (laughs)' and when he returned he tried to be careful: 'The clothes that I would wear … I would wash them after my visit, I'd put my shoes into a plastic bag … I'd have a shower first and then go into my room.' His family members 'were a little apprehensive at first and then they realised that… well, anyone can die at any given point.' Eventually, the whole family caught the virus:

I caught the virus a long time after the initial wave … I caught it towards the end of the second wave … All of a sudden my eldest daughter began coughing and she went to test … I was out shopping at the time and when I got home, my third daughter is quite animated and she said: 'Dad, before you do anything, you need to get tested'. And when we tested at home, we were negative … but when I went to get tested at Watney Market test centre, we were all tested and we received the results a day later … We were all positive.

2.8 Family Dynamics and Generation

So, the dynamics within families clearly emerged as a key theme during the interviews. Irfan Iqbal chose to place these dynamics within the broader context of different generations when he discussed the issue of vaccine hesitancy:

> *What we saw was a lot of elderly people who are fearful, actually, because my mum is elderly … but it's the younger generation, and a lot of them influencing the parents saying: … 'Don't take the vaccine' … And we had that sort of big, big argument in the community going on … But all the while … elderly people who are isolating, [are] thinking, you know: 'Let me just go out and see [my family]' … because a lot of older people probably lived with one or two other kids. But the other children isolated from them and … just had them on the phone … and obviously, they couldn't see their grandchildren.*

He proceeded to claim that communication between family members about observing official regulations even when they interfered with the ritual calendar was more powerful than top-down messages from the state:

> *I think those messages are more strong than the government … because people who speak from personal experience … especially if it's someone from your family … they're likely to listen to them more … And I've seen families … parts of families, who tell family members: … 'No, we're not going to have a big feast this year because of Covid and everyone has to stay away.' And it takes one or two in the family to be strong and spread that message … and say: 'We're not going to do this, this year as we did all these years ago because let's just not, because something could happen because we've been silly.'*

Plans to celebrate weddings, for example, had to be reorganised, even if some people hoped to circumvent the restrictions in the case of small events. As Irfan Iqbal also commented, during the first lockdown those, who were 'having not large weddings,' sought to 'flout the rules … trying to find places or restaurants who open their basements for a smaller wedding and stuff.'

2.9 State Regulations and Muslim Funerals

At the beginning of the 2020 lockdown the central government discussed introducing legislation, which would provide legal support for the measures it was considering to counter the pandemic. One of the most controversial elements of the proposed legislation was:

a section that would have given local authorities the power to cremate the bodies of coronavirus victims without consent, and "streamlining" the process by removing the need for a medical certificate to do so—something expressly illegal in the UK since 1961.[11]

As this news report commented:

Such legislation would have put the government at odds not only with the families of victims who may oppose such a move, but also with several religious groups, including the UK's Muslim and Jewish communities, as cremation is not permitted as a form of burial in either faith.

Muslim and Jewish representative bodies successfully campaigned against the cremation proposal at the national level but it clearly antagonised Muslims and Jews at the local level as Afia Begum, a Bangladeshi Muslim funeral director, recalled when she was interviewed in November 2021:

The Muslim community were up in arms because they felt really, really threatened because they thought that their loved ones were going to be cremated because the (Coronavirus) Act allowed this. It's the government that comes in and the government decides to run funerals with the army ... they were going to take over all the funerals ... Then it would have meant that they could've done what they wanted regardless of your background or your wishes. It's so important to get the funeral right ... And so people campaigned. We wrote letters in support and in against the government being able to do that.

Afia Begum's parents lived in a predominantly Bangladeshi neighbourhood near Spitalfields but Afia moved to a more culturally diverse area of the borough as an adult before settling in a neighbouring borough further east where she had raised three children. She was a co-director of a small funeral company that served a culturally diverse area where Bangladeshis constituted only a small proportion of the population. However, her continuing links with Tower Hamlets and Bangladeshi background meant that when the pandemic struck, many Bangladeshi families sought her emotional support and professional expertise.

She tried to bend the official rules once the first lockdown ended in the name of compassion. When the government formally allowed people to meet others at a distance in small groups—'the rule of six'—she took as

[11] https://www.arabnews.com/node/1647241/world, accessed 25/6/2023.

many mourners as possible to the cemetery so that they could take videos of the proceedings to send to relatives and friends within the UK and abroad, particularly Bangladesh:

> *A lot of the funerals that were allowed were secretly being video'd because in the early days, only six people were allowed. … One of the Muslim cemeteries, they were really, really strict and so they would only allow six people. I thought we can take two more people because in our vehicle … I pretended that two of the family were my staff. And then they caught in with it… and they said: 'Oh no … you can't do that' … But it was like at least I tried … And I did that a few times and I got away with it. But the point is that you have a go. And then they were saying: "No filming" … so they would put their phone in their top pocket and they caught onto that as well.*

When the second lockdown was introduced during the autumn of 2021, the officials at this cemetery had reluctantly become more flexible:

> *I think [the Muslim cemetery] got a lot of criticism from the community for being so [strict] … They became a bit softer but because they became softer, they allowed so many people into the funeral for the burial … and I could see it wasn't in their values … because their values are being strict.*

However, other Muslim cemeteries were much more relaxed: 'You have another Muslim cemetery and they're like: "Yeah, anything goes, as long as everything's done, the paperwork's done, the finances are done" … They interpreted what they wanted.' As Afia concluded: 'So we had these two extremes … and again I felt that we have to be compassionate here.'

Mourning is a complex social and cultural process and the experiences that follow death are often multidimensional (Silverman et al., 2021). In the pandemic, however, it became a solitary gesture. Often, religious figures acted as guides and teachers to facilitate what was often an unfamiliar process for individuals who had lost loved ones because of the virus. Many people did not know the religious and cultural rites and practices that need to be followed in order to ensure a 'good death' (Islam, 2023; Gatrad, 1994). As one of our interlocutors explained:

> *There were instances, as I'm sure you know, where the father passed away very suddenly and the child had never had to experience death in this way or deal with a dead body in this way, it was a first for the family … In Bangladesh or*

here in normal times, when someone passes away, everyone comes to the deceased's house and comforts the family but we had a family here where the children did not know what to do because their father was the first to die in this way, he had died in the hospital and they didn't know what to do or where to go ... This is not somebody's daily routine and it was very sudden ... People suffered immensely because of this...

Mourning together is part of Bangladeshi culture and people's networks provide crucial support at these times (Gardner, 1998, 2002, 2009). Comfort is given in various ways, emotionally and physically. People often bring food to the deceased's family, make arrangements for their welfare and offer words of comfort; support is offered mostly by friends and family during this time (Spruyt, 1999). Before the pandemic local social networks were crucial in helping the bereaved understand and partake in rituals as well as cope with bureaucratic issues since many Bangladeshi elders died in hospitals and hospices. During the pandemic lockdown, communal comfort was prohibited and the telephone became the key instrument which enabled people to collectively mourn. Local networks became crucial to helping Bangladeshis in Tower Hamlets negotiate with official NHS structures and other institutions involved in the process of death and dying, such as funeral services.

Arun Chowdhury, whom we met earlier in the chapter, used the death of Prince Philip, Queen Elizabeth's husband, in April 2021 as an example of a 'good death':

When Prince Philip died, there was an announcement that he died peacefully surrounded by his family ... Have you noticed that? That notice has been given by Buckingham Palace, the highest authority of the United Kingdom ... That is their belief ... when people die, they want to see their family in front of them ... That is the example of the peaceful dying.

The many 'bad deaths' that occurred during the pandemic where people died alone in hospital and their infected bodies had to be very carefully processed before and during the funeral led some people at least to see the virus as a curse. As one interlocutor commented:

They see Corona as some sort of curse because why people said when they died, people can't touch the body ... it's some sort of degraded thing ... Even your family cannot touch you; your family cannot go near you at the funeral.

Another interlocutor not only referred to the belief in a curse but also raised the issue of shame:

> *I want to die with my family surrounding me … but people said this virus is a curse … Those who died in winter 2020, death was very terrible and people tried to hide the shame of dying from Corona … because it was seen as a curse towards [the] family.*

2.10 A Wider Community: Middle-Class Residents

Although our research has focused on the relationship between the state and local residents in terms of the Bangladeshi Muslim population, Tower Hamlets contained people from a variety of social, cultural and economic backgrounds. As the first section of this chapter made clear, the development of 'Docklands' as a banking and financial services centre has led to the settlement of middle-class professionals in what was a predominantly working class area. One of our interlocutors, Irfan Iqbal, was not only a Labour Party councillor but was employed by the Canary Wharf Group in Docklands as a community outreach worker so he was in a good position to comment on the class divisions within the borough as well as how middle-class professionals sought to engage across ethnic and class differences.

> *So this area obviously has a rich history about it and how people have moved from poverty… and so you've got one of the biggest global city estates and then you have estates where people are living in poverty and it's all around Tower Hamlets because you've got the City side … The reality is that you've got a lot of people who are vulnerable and have low paid jobs and have large families and there's overcrowded housing and all that stuff … So there's a big gap in what one person earns to another … There's a huge divide.*

Yet because mobility was restricted during the pandemic, middle-class residents were encouraged to engage more with their locality and work with other from different socio-economic and cultural backgrounds. As Irfan Iqbal noted:

> *In my ward and other places we had covid community groups that were set up and every week we saw numbers increasing and people were coming up and they were professionals and people were saying that: 'Actually, we've never been part of the community and I want to help. What do I do?' … It's not just people from*

one faith or one community ... there was a whole spectrum of people coming together ... They probably couldn't go to their parents' home because their parents were isolating in the country somewhere, so they only place they could be was at home and being at home for seven days is not a nice place to be ... You want to go out and when you can't you think ... the only thing I can do is help my community ... There were adverts on the estate boards saying if you want to help and you're not isolating, contact us through this number.

2.11 Conclusion

This chapter has explored the relationship between the state and Bangladeshi Muslims in the London borough of Tower Hamlets by first outlining the measures taken by the state when the pandemic struck in 2020 and then focusing on how Bangladeshis themselves reacted. Our qualitative study examined the important role played by Bangladeshi activists at the meso level between the macro level of the state and the micro level of people's everyday lives. In order to reveal what happened during 2020 and 2021 'on the ground,' we also contacted those who were not engaged in community activism.

The qualitative data enabled us to explore the different ways in which the activists contributed to the meso level between the state and Bangladeshi citizens in the borough. They drew on the political and community networks which have developed over the last forty years as Bangladeshis became the dominant force in local politics. These networks helped them to combat the considerable scepticism about government advice, which was weakened by disagreements between them and scientists and distrust towards big business who were often seen as taking advantage of the emergency.

The interviews with both these 'experts' and the 'non-experts' also illustrated the economic problems caused by the government's restrictions for families, which relied on members having to go out to work, as well as the various ways in which state regulations were observed and the importance placed on 'playing the game' even when state regulations disrupted the Muslim ritual calendar. The interviews also raised the issue of trust in relation to the state and the different ways in which public institutions such as cemeteries interpreted state regulations; the part played by funeral directors in bending the rules in order to show compassion to the bereaved, as well as the importance of digital communications in facilitating the flow of information and images between the locality and the wider world, especially Bangladesh, and the issue of digital exclusion. Some of the data also raised the issue of people's reaction to the virus as a curse and feelings of shame around death caused by the virus. Finally, the support provided by middle-class residents of the borough emphasised the importance of looking beyond the Bangladeshi community to wider definitions of community. During the restrictions on mobility in 2020 and early 2021, residents were encouraged by the force of circumstances to look beyond the divisions of ethnicity and class and help one another to cope with a health emergency that posed a threat to everyone.

References

Alexander, C. (2011). Making Bengali Brick Lane: Claiming and Contesting Space in East London. *British Journal of Sociology, 62*(2), 201–220. https://doi.org/10.1111/j.1468-4446.2011.01361.x

Ansari, H. (2011). *The Making of the East London Mosque, 1910–1951: Minutes of the London Mosque Fund and East London Mosque Trust Ltd.* Cambridge University Press for the Royal Historical Society.

Ansari, H. (2013). 'A Mosque in London Worthy of the Tradition of Islam and Worthy of the Capital of the British Empire': The Struggle to Create Muslim Space, 1910–1944. In S. Nasta (Ed.), *India in Britain* (pp. 80–95). Palgrave Macmillan. https://doi.org/10.1057/9780230392724_6

Brownhill, S. (2010). London Docklands Revisited: The Dynamics of Waterfront Development. In G. Desfor et al. (Eds.), *Transforming Urban Waterfronts: Fixity and Flow* (pp. 121–142). Routledge.

Butler, T. (2007). Re-urbanizing London Docklands: Gentrification, Suburbanization or New Urbanism? *International Journal of Urban and Regional Research, 31*(4), 759–781. https://doi.org/10.1111/j.1468-2427.2007.00758.x

Carey, S., & Shukur, A. (1985). A Profile of the Bangladeshi Community in East London. *New Community, 12*(3), 405–417. https://doi.org/10.1080/1369183X.1985.9975918

Eade, J. (1989). *The Politics of Community.* Avebury.

Eade, J. (2000). *Placing London: From Imperial Capital to Global City.* Berghahn Books.

Gardner, K. (1998). Death, Burial and Bereavement Amongst Bengali Muslims in Tower Hamlets, East London. *Journal of Ethnic and Migration Studies, 24*(3), 507–521. https://doi.org/10.1080/1369183X.1998.9976647

Gardner, K. (2002). Death of a Migrant: Transnational Death Rituals and Gender among British Sylhetis. *Global Networks, 2*(3), 191–204. https://doi.org/10.1111/1471-0374.00036

Gardner, K. (2009). Lives in Motion: The Life-Course, Movement and Migration in Bangladesh. *Journal of South Asian Development, 4*(2), 229–251. https://doi.org/10.1177/097317410900400204

Gatrad, A. (1994). Muslim Customs Surrounding Death, Bereavement, Postmortem Examinations, and Organ Transplants. *British Medical Journal, 309*, 521. https://doi.org/10.1136/bmj.309.6953.521

Glynn, S. (2016). *Class, Ethnicity and Religion in the Bengali East End: A Political History*. Manchester University Press.

Islam, F. (2023). Pandemic-induced Deathscapes: End-of-life, Funerary and Bereavement Challenges for British-Bangladeshi Muslims. *Social & Cultural Geography, 24*(3–4), 409–427. https://doi.org/10.1080/14649365.2022.2130416

Platt, L., & Warwick, R. (2020). *Are Some Ethnic Groups More Vulnerable To COVID-19 Than Others?* Institute for Fiscal Studies. https://ifs.org.uk/sites/default/files/output_url_files/Are-some-ethnic-groups-more-vulnerable-to%252520COVID-19-than-others-V2-IFS-Briefing-Note.pdf

Silverman, G. S., Baroiller, A., & Hemer, S. R. (2021). Culture and Grief: Ethnographic Perspectives on Ritual, Relationships and Remembering. *Death Studies, 45*(1), 1–8. https://doi.org/10.1080/07481187.2020.1851885

Spruyt, O. (1999). Community-based Palliative Care for Bangladeshi Patients in East London. *Accounts of Bereaved Carers. Palliative medicine, 13*(2), 119–129. https://doi.org/10.1191/026921699667569476

CHAPTER 3

Turkish Migration in Stuttgart: Potential and Limits of 'Integrationism'

Jörg Dürrschmidt

3.1 Migration and Integration in Germany: A Society in Transition

German society can be regarded as a society in transition as far as issues of migration/integration are concerned. While this society has a long history of migration, mainly involving those seeking work and asylum, it has only recently started to face up to the reality of being a country of immigration. The concept that best captures this shift was coined by a migration/integration scholar who herself has family roots elsewhere: 'Post-Migration Society' (Foroutan, 2015). This term refers to the fact that migration has irrevocably become part of everyday life in Germany, where approximately one-third of the population has a migration experience of some kind that acts as a familial reference point. Migration is here to stay—it is not an exceptional phenomenon or something that should place society in a state

J. Dürrschmidt (✉)
Ludwigsburg University of Applied Sciences (HVF), Ludwigsburg, Germany
e-mail: joerg.duerrschmidt@hs-ludwigsburg.de

M. Caselli et al. (eds.), *Migrants' (Im)mobilities in Three European Urban Contexts*, Europe in a Global Context,
https://doi.org/10.1007/978-3-031-53773-8_3

of emergency. Consequently, society as a whole—from everyday culture to state institutions—has to open up and adapt to this new normal of (im) migration.

This change has three main implications. Firstly, integration efforts have to be mobilized by all parties involved. While previously integration was mainly seen as an effort required from the migrant, research shows that it should be seen as a two-way process. However, as far as the general public is concerned, an Established/Outsider pattern of thinking still prevails. From this perspective the onus of integration lies on those migrating rather than by the society integrating them. Secondly, a post-migrant society has to close the 'gaps in representation' within its institutional setup, i.e. from representational bodies in the realm of politics right up to role models in the media. At the moment migrants are largely underrepresented in politics, media, higher education, and public administration, to name just a few areas which require a renegotiation of opportunity and access. Thirdly, the new heterogeneous Germany needs a fresh narrative that presents migration as normal rather than as exceptional within a static society. In order to also symbolically integrate the 'new Germans', German post-migrant society has been looking (in vain) towards North America (the USA and Canada), without really finding (as yet) an equivalent to the 'American way of life' narrative that collectively binds society beyond a legal or constitutional sense.

Some other-related concepts have developed out of the controversial discourse concerning integration. On the more conservative side of the political spectrum this search for a new narrative about shared values has been (re)linked to the idea of a *Leitkultur* or a 'guiding culture', while the discourse leaning more towards the political Left has answered *Leitkultur* with *Leitbild*, i.e. 'image of a concrete utopia' where German society can act as an open society fit for the twenty-first century (Williams, 2014; Foroutan, 2015a).

This political debate reflects the ambiguous impact of European multilevel governance on migration and integration governance and policy. Intense policy uploading and downloading between the EU, national, and regional-cum-municipal levels has led to changes in the realm of integration politics and policy too. It has been argued that sub-state political units have become more empowered and involved in migration policy, in general, and migrant integration policies, in particular (Hepburn & Zapata-Barrero, 2014, p. 4). Whether this amounts to a sustainable 'local turn' in migrant integration policy—with benefits for the societal standing of migrant communities—remains open for debate (Schönwälder, 2020, p. 3).

Some observers have claimed that there has also been a 'national turn on local integration policy' (Emilsson, 2015, p. 2). This change reflects a change of societal climate after 9/11 as well as neoliberal austerity politics which have resulted in a more centralized control of public services in many European societies (Galandini et al., 2019; Emilsson, 2015; Campomori & Caponio, 2017; Green, 2007). Hence, Germany introduced a comprehensive national integration plan during 2005 that emphasized a relationship of compliance between the state and migrant populations, which was mainly based on mainstreaming integration measures and a civic value discourse (Williams, 2014, p. 67f.).

To some extent this development resonated in academic debates, insofar as there has been a revitalized interest on the intersection of migration policy with issues of trust and social capital. Social cohesion, it is argued, needs mutual trust amongst individuals but also between the state and its people. Trust, in turn, is based on familiarity as a shared sense of normality in everyday life. Such a sense of social cohesion, the argument continues, is a crucial precondition for successfully integrating newcomers, while the arrival of too many newcomers would undermine this trust-based sense of coherence (Münkler, 2018).

In this regard it is noteworthy that the peculiarity of German migration as predominantly 'guestworker' migration has more than elsewhere led to an accentuation of the division between society and nation or, for that matter, between structural and cultural integration. While the state as the guardian of liberal order safeguards for all residents access to economic opportunity and welfare based on their economic contribution, the same state ensures that these residential rights remain detached from an ethnocentrically defined national community (Joppke, 2004, p. 452). The handling of access to citizenship in its narrower and wider meaning is of crucial importance here. While access to legal citizenship might have been liberalized through the 1999 Nationality Act, which saw the introduction of *jus soli* elements, the distribution of social respect and everyday cultural recognition as the essential fabric of moral citizenship outlasted these formal changes and still tends to work according to the principle of *jus sanguinis* (Geißler, 2004, p. 288; Schönwälder & Triadafilopoulos, 2012).

Accordingly, some commentators have detected a 'paradigm shift' in German integration policy between 2000 and 2010. This view is based on the change within public discourse and the political elite from denial to acceptance that Germany has become a country of immigration (Williams, 2014). However, other commentators tend to see a 'path dependency' working underneath the liberalization tendencies in integration policy (Green, 2007, p. 96). They claim that the citizenship reforms serve to perpetuate a long-lasting structure of the 'established and outsiders' based on the prerogative of 'ethnocentricity', even if disguised by a partly open allegiance to a 'community of value' (Lewicki, 2018, pp. 501, 506). Those fully belonging to the 'imagined community' of the nation enjoy 'moral citizenship' as opposed to and also superior to 'formal citizenship' (van Campenhout & van Houtum, 2021, p. 8ff.). The reintroduction in 2008 of citizenship tests next to language exams for those applying for German citizenship is an indicator of the guarding of the national community against 'untrustworthy and threatening outsiders'. According to this logic of cultural exclusion if these formal impediments do not work, one could then draw on the 'less tangible but perhaps even more important symbolic cues addressed to immigrants by members of the host society' (Schönwälder & Triadafilopoulos, 2012, pp. 52, 57, 61).

Thus, the discourse of 'formal and moral deservedness' of belonging was well established at the eve of the Covid-19 pandemic and was awaiting its litmus test (van Campenhout & van Houtum, 2021, p. 1). Therefore, it should not come as a surprise that these measures of guarding formal and moral belonging to German society were primarily directed towards people with Turkish roots, since they are the largest single group amongst Germany's migrant population and they figure strongly amongst those applying for naturalization. At the same time, unlike 'elite migrants' from EU countries, given their Muslim background they are perceived as less trustworthy in terms of 'genuine acceptance of liberal democratic norms' (Schönwälder & Triadafilopoulos, 2012, pp. 58f., 62; Lewicki, 2018). Some have pointed to the paradox that while 'German public opinion includes some of the deepest anti-Muslim sentiments in Europe' over the last decades, 'Muslims in Germany have become more economically and educationally successful and more integrated into social and cultural life than is commonly assumed' (Foroutan, 2013, p. 1).

3.2 Migration and Integration in Stuttgart: Assembly Line Integration

The New York Times feature titled 'Stuttgart Struggles to House the Migrants It Embraces' (Kimmelmann, 2015) captures quite well the ambiguities of local migrant integration in the capital of the Baden-Württemberg region. As the powerhouse of a booming region, it cannot but be a city of integration. Labour migrants have been the engine of industrial growth and ongoing post-industrial transformation. Bosch, Porsche, and Mercedes rely on the import of skilled and (although today less so) unskilled labour and brain power to remain the prime symbols of 'made in Germany'. Quite aptly, *The NYT* describes Stuttgart's social DNA as 'gear box assembly line integration'.

Yet, this mode of integration is not the same as the 'tolerant, assimilative cosmopolitanism' of a global city (Eade 2000, p. 4). Stuttgart, just like Germany as a whole, has for a long time heavily relied on the integrating power of the work place. It was assumed that being employed equalled being integrated and everything else was left to the semi-private sphere of the neighbourhood. Here, despite housing people from more than 170 nations, Stuttgart differs from a global city like London. Instead of 'live and let life', the guiding principle for newcomers has always been a rather brazen law of local/regional everyday order centred around the custom of 'Kehrwoche' (lit. sweeping week). While on the surface it means doing your weekly contribution towards an orderly city by keeping your stairs, pavement, and courtyard clean and tidy, it is the signifier of a fine-grained everyday culture of mutual recognition and observation that offers you a strict choice: blend in or become a frowned upon outsider. Still today many of its inhabitants describe Stuttgart (in most instances lovingly) as a 'large village' rather than a metropolis. Thus, *The NYT*'s description of the city's mode of integration as 'melting pot urbanism' kind of fits the bill, although its driving force is the assembly line and an observant neighbourhood, i.e. not the kind of public encounter and 'ethos of mixing' attributed to a genuine metropolis (Wessendorf, 2013). Stuttgart appears to be an 'orthogenetic' rather than 'heterogenetic' city to borrow Hannerz's (1998, p. 127) useful distinction.

Unlike other German industrial cities Stuttgart already saw its first peak of labour migration during the 1960s. It all started with 300 Italians in 1955, who were recruited to work in the agricultural outskirts of Stuttgart and who later moved into the city's brick factories. They were followed by labour migrants from Greece, Turkey, Portugal, and former Yugoslavia. By 1970 Stuttgart was the first and only city in Germany with more than 12% 'foreigners' amongst its population, increasing to 17% in the 1980s. Stuttgart was also a trendsetter amongst German cities when it launched in 1983 the first 'immigration committee' (Ausländerausschuss), which was then adopted as a general consultative body in most German cities with migrant populations (Meier-Braun, 2009).

Meanwhile, a broad network of heterogeneous organizations has emerged in Stuttgart representing migrant life in the city and engaging in dialogue with and participating in local politics. For instance, there is the Stuttgart Council of Religions, established in 2015, with a roll-on mode of formal leadership. Between 2019 and 2021, a representative of *DITIB* (Turkish-Islamic Union for Religious Affairs) served as head (coordinator) of this interreligious forum. *DITIB* is symbolically important as the Turkish Muslim community has been the steady focus of integration politics and policy in Stuttgart. Already in 1999 the 'German-Turkish Forum' was launched by its mayor, Wolfgang Schuster. This organization was always intended to be more than merely a forum for symbolic dialogue; it operated educational programmes and provided mentorships and scholarships, all of which were designed to facilitate cultural integration through individual upward social mobility.

Amongst Stuttgart's integration policy actors, the role of charismatic mayors cannot be overestimated. Paraphrasing Barber's (2013) bestseller *If Mayors Ruled the World*, we could answer the related question 'what if mayors made (im)migration policy?' by looking at Stuttgart as a good case in point. Manfred Rommel, who governed the city from 1974 to 1996, introduced quite early the term 'multicultural society' into local political discourse, even though as a Christian Democrat he was located at the rather conservative end of party politics. For him the term was simply a description of the lived reality of his city and a precondition for its sustainable economic growth (Meier-Braun, 2009, p. 371f.).

His successor, Wolfgang Schuster—another member of the Christian Democrat party and, indeed, one of the mayors portrayed in Barber's book—developed the Stuttgart Model further through a pragmatic and utilitarian approach towards (im)migration. He established the aforementioned integration policy unit, attached it to his mayoral office, and promoted the Stuttgart Alliance for Integration (*Stuttgarter Bündnis für Integration*). One could say he modernized Stuttgart's integration policy through a 'mainstreaming' approach (ibid. 373f.). Thus, when the Green politician, Fritz Kuhn, took over the mayor's office in 2013, the field was already paved for a liberal and welcoming (im)migration policy that would fit the Green Party's agenda.

Hence, it could be argued that despite its less glamourous and more utilitarian focus on guest worker migration, Stuttgart's integration policy has successfully contributed to a culturally diversified—not quite the same as diverse—city (Diehl & Schieckoff, 2021, p. 35f.). Stuttgart has quite early recognized labour migration not just as an engine of growth in a narrow economic sense but also as a seedbed of innovation in more general terms. *The New York Times* article claims that Stuttgart has now the highest percentage of entrepreneurs from a migrant background (see also Statistisches Amt LHS, 2014). Moreover, many migrants have moved into hospitality and thereby contribute to Stuttgart having increasingly less the feel of a 'large village'.

Yet, looking more deeply at the reality of 'guest worker' integration, the situation is more complicated. Reflecting Stuttgart's mode of 'ambivalent integration' outlined earlier in this chapter, despite structural integration through an efficient placement within employment, the pattern of integration could be described as marginalized cultural integration. This marginalization is partly offset by a strong emotional attachment to neighbourhood and city district. However, this local attachment involves small (in terms of extension) and homogeneous (in terms of social mixing) networks that patronize the local neighbourhood but hardly venture outside, leading to tendencies towards the spatial segmentation of migrant youth, in particular (Albrecht & Reschl, 2005, p. 75ff.). Similarly, the city's elaborate fabric of consultative bodies concerned with migrant integration is ambiguous. They can forcefully articulate migrant aspiration in local politics and policy but at the same time they tend to lack democratic legitimacy and real political impact. Rather than challenging the status quo of local integration policy, these bodies cream off ethno-cultural elites and have been criticized as constituting an 'institutional ghetto' (Guentner & Stanton, 2013).

Nieswand's (2021) concept of 'integrationism' is useful to understanding this ambivalent pattern of integration. Drawing on empirical research into integration policy within Baden-Württemberg, the region of which Stuttgart is the centre, Nieswand describes the policy as a quasi-ideological 'bridging frame' (ibid., p. 89) that legitimates actors involved in policy coalitions between the state and non-state actors. Drawing on the work of Charles Taylor, Nieswand argues that when a society considers 'integration' as a 'hypergood', it generates 'frameworks of strong evaluation' (ibid., p. 84). However, because harsh reality seldom matches the abstract ideal of integration, it is often complemented by 'techno-administrative' action (ibid., p. 86). Hence, where the inclusion of migrant populations into the educational or health care system, for example, is weak, rather than challenging established social disparities between mainstream and migrant population 'integrationism', as a mode of governance, falls back on technical and administrative procedures.

3.3 Turkish Migrants in Stuttgart

According to figures by the 'Micro Census' survey from the German Federal Statistical Office, in 2021 there were around 22.3 million people with a so-called migration background living in Germany. This corresponds to 27.2% of the overall population of Germany. By comparison, in 2020 this proportion was at 26.7%. A little more than half of the people with a 'migration background' are German passport holders. Amongst Germany's population with a 'migration background', 12.3% or 2,750,000 with roots in Turkey are the largest group. In keeping with the overall tendency, about half of this group are German passport holders, while it is estimated that 285,000 hold dual citizenship (https://mediendienst-integration.de/english/facts-figures.html [23.07. 2023]).

There is, as elsewhere in Europe, a pull towards the big cities, with some 43% of those with a migration background living in urban areas such as Stuttgart, where the proportion of migrants has increased from 36% in 1999 to 45% in 2019 and 45% of these hold a German passport. In sum, many of those formally registered with a 'migration background' were actually born and or have been socialized in Germany (Diehl & Schieckoff, 2021, p. 34).

By the end of 2018 (*Stuttgarter Zeitung* Feb. 18, 2019; https://www.domino1.stuttgart.de/web/komunis/komunissde.nsf) Stuttgart had 614,365 inhabitants and it is expected to have 650,000 inhabitants by 2030. The proportion of those with a 'migration background' has reached 45.3% and people with roots in Turkey (ca. 34,000), Italy (18,000), Croatia (15,000), and Greece (13,000) still form the most substantial migrant groups. However, the numbers of migrants from Syria and Iraq (both above 5000) as well as from India and China have also substantially increased (all in the ballpark of 4000–5000) and have now reached a similar size to the smaller established migrant communities from Serbia, Spain, or Portugal. Thus, despite a certain diversification of incoming migration, in terms of sheer numbers, the Turkish community in Stuttgart that has emerged mainly in the wake of 'guest worker migration' has been and still is of major significance.

One reason to take a stricter approach towards integration was the fear that the 'guest worker' milieu would develop into a persistent 'ethclass' with undertones of 'parallel lives' (Geißler, 2004, p. 288f.). However, as commonly assumed for immigrant settlement structure in Germany in general (Schönwälder & Söhn, 2009), Stuttgart's built environment and infrastructural setup do not lend itself to outright 'ghettoization'. However, in 2012 (Siedentop and Fina) Stuttgart Council discussed, based on statistical data, long-term tendencies towards 'a new geography of segregation', since gentrification and disparities in wealth have led to migrants moving disproportionately from the inner city to the outskirts, leading to 'larger and coherent quarters with ethnic dominance' in boroughs such as Feuerbach and Zuffenhausen. Next to the inner borough of Bad Cannstatt, it is in these boroughs that we would find 'ethnically mixed immigrant neighbourhoods' (Schönwälder & Söhn, 2009, p. 1446) as well as the largest population of Turkish origin (Landeshauptstadt Stuttgart Statistisches Amt, 2020; see Fig. 3.1, where the reddish colouring indicates overrepresentation and greenish colour shows the opposite).

As is often the case, the key to understanding the logic of integration is not so much found in numbers but symbols and every day discourse. Although there might be a stronger numerical presence of Turkish life in boroughs such as Bad Cannstatt, Feuerbach is widely seen as more important. People, whom you talk to on the streets in Feuerbach, describe the Turkish quarter as 'little Istanbul', the 'Turkish Ghetto', or 'Stuttgart's bazaar'. The best description perhaps has been coined by a journalist of

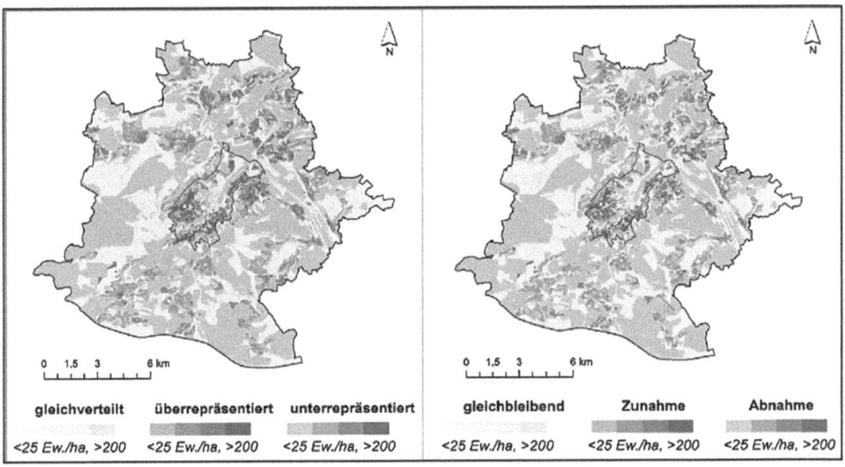

Fig. 3.1 Location quotient for people with Turkish migration background, comparison: 1999 to 2010. (Source: Siedentop & Fina, 2012; www.stuttgart.de/item/show/16332/1/publ/21571)

the *Stuttgarter Nachrichten* (18.12. 2015; https://www.stuttgarter-nachrichten.de/inhalt.tuerkisches-viertel-in-feuerbach-grosser-basar-in-alten-werkshallen.90763667-bebd-4d57-a632-4a9acd19fe49.html [20.05. 2021]), who described it as an 'ethnic outlet'. Here you can find most exotic fruits, herbs, vegetables, and so on which are not available in normal supermarkets, and you can find furniture, wedding dresses, interior design, jewellery, and even books that do not cater to the average 'Stuttgarter'. You will also find other services such as a hair dressing salon, a flight agency, a café selling Turkish sweets, and much more.

This Turkish neighbourhood actually comprises no more than a couple of streets next to the railway. It is the child of structural change in industrial Stuttgart where the last stakeholder of the industrial age—a car supplier—finally closed its outlets in 2011. In 1993 a mosque was launched here under the umbrella of *DITIB* (short for: Turkish-Islamic Union for Religious Affairs) and Turkish life began to move into the quarter. Yet even today it is not the largest Turkish neighbourhood, because it is still a mixed district of business, services, and housing. However, the *DITIB* mosque has become the hub of Turkish life in Stuttgart. It currently has a catchment area of 1200 and there is a plan to redevelop it to cater for around 5000 people (source: interviews; Fig. 3.2).

The *DITIB* mosque is not the only mosque in town but will be the largest in south-west Germany, and more than the current mosque, it will be a centre of social and cultural community life. Under the officially

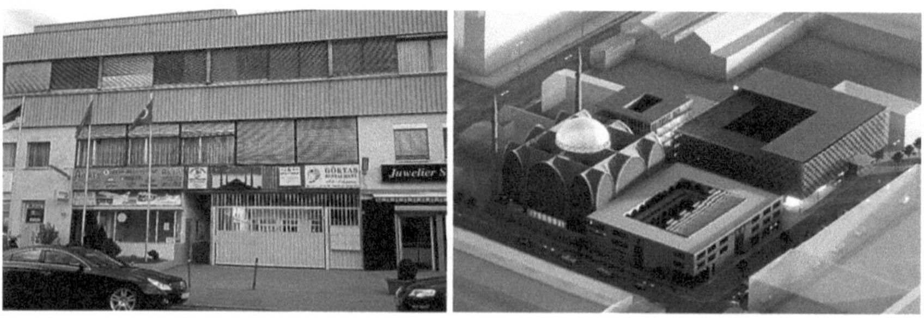

Fig. 3.2 Old and new mosque building in Stuttgart Feuerbach. (Source: https://www.feuerbach.de/historie/begehbares-feuerbacher-gedaechtnis/moschee; https://www.stuttgarter-zeitung.de/inhalt.mauserstrasse-in-stuttgart-feuerbach-entwuerfe-fuer-eine-neue-moschee-vorgestellt.73699505-3b40-40df-8b90-95d642af9d82.html [20.05.2021])

approved plan 70% of the space will be used for social functions (from education to recreation). As usual with mosque developments here and elsewhere in Europe, there was a dispute about the height of the minaret (initially envisaged at 27 metres). Notably, around 2014/2015 at the height of the planning process a heated discussion took place that was mainly driven by the right wing-populist citizen initiative 'Pax Europe' (Bürgerbewegung Pax Europa—*BPE*), which is close to the larger *PEGIDA* (short for: Patriotic Europeans Against the Islamization of the West).

As always with buildings of high symbolic significance, they are subject to different interpretations. The real issue in this case seems to be the visibility of Turkish Muslim culture in Stuttgart's public everyday life. Some see this as a positive commitment about staying and regarding Stuttgart as home. Others fear that mosques represent the Islamization of urban life in a city with approximately 10% Muslim population, of which 75% have Turkish roots (Frisoli & Mäding, 2019). A sober analysis would perhaps say that, either way, these are reactions to the new social self-confidence of the 'advancing stranger' (Hüttermann, 2000).

The borough council of Stuttgart Feuerbach remained and remains remarkably relaxed about it all. They point to the long-standing interpersonal trust relationship they have developed since 1993 with the organizers of the Feuerbach Mosque (for more detail about the local policy implications, see Chap. 8).

3.4 The Corona Pandemic in Germany and Its Impact on the Migrant Population: An Overview

Many outside-observers believe that the German government, in general, and health governance, in particular, have handled the pandemic rather well compared with other European countries (Hanson et al., 2021). They mention the fine-grained balance between diversity and inclusiveness within the federal system, the effective engagement between politics and science in managing uncertainty, and the role of the media and, in particular, the evening talk show format. Together these factors helped to generate public support and transmit relevant information as well as a policy narrative and, finally, the resulting broad societal support which, only at the end of the pandemic, started to waver. It seems that the preparedness of those in charge for 'repeated communication of uncertainty … made it substantially easier to adapt messages in time', and generated societal trust and resilience that only 'hit its limits at the third wave' when the 'patchwork quilt' of regionalized and partly even localized Covid-19 measures outstretched people's compliance (ibid., pp. 1, 7, 11f.).

As far as the timeline of the pandemic and the response to it is concerned, they follow roughly the rhythms as found elsewhere in Europe (for the following section, see ibid., p. 3f. and in more detail: https://www.bundesgesundheitsministerium.de/coronavirus/chronik-coronavirus.html). At the end of January 2020 Germany detected its first cases of SARS-CoV-2 and when in March Germany went in its first lockdown this was an acknowledgement that there was an internal transmission of what was initially perceived as an external threat. Subsequently, public life came more or less to a standstill and many families got used to distant learning and internet-based working from home. In May 2020 the Covid-19 restrictions were relaxed and an almost normal summer followed, based on the responsible wearing of face masks and the use of a Coronavirus tracing app. During autumn, however, a second Covid-19 wave with new variants hit the country, which led to a new 'circuit breaker' in November and then a 'partial' lockdown in December.

Around the beginning of 2021 the vaccination programme began starting with the elderly and frontline workers (health care and care for the elderly). February 2021 saw the reopening of schools, only for a third lockdown to be implemented in April after considerable public dispute about legitimacy and efficiency. Covid-19 prevention measures within the federal system were then increasingly decentralized with the emphasis shifting from prevention to management of the epidemic. From July an EU digital Covid-19 vaccination certificate was rolled out which enabled those vaccinated to travel around Europe during the summer and was used to control access to public venues, for example. Nevertheless, in December 2021 restrictions were tightened again in order to overcome the fourth (Omicron) wave.

Almost routinely, February 2022 saw once more the relaxation of restrictions but this was followed by intense public debate about the introduction of mandatory vaccinations—a proposal that was eventually rejected by the German Bundestag during April when most of the restrictions were abolished. Subsequently, the Corona pandemic faded and the ending of the requirement to wear mask on public transport on 2 February 2023 marked the symbolic end of the pandemic in Germany.

The pandemic in 2020 hit a German society that was sensitized to the ambivalences of 'integration', as described in Sect. 3.1 of this chapter, as well as to the emergent discourse of identity politics. However, what it lacked was the experience of managing a multi-cultural society with ethnic minority populations like other European countries, such as the UK. Consequently, there was a certain hesitancy about addressing the identity of migrants in terms of ethnic identity. As a result, there is not much statistical data about the 'likely disproportionate impact on immigrants' by Covid-19 (OECD, 2020). For instance, there is no data available for Germany's migrant population concerning infection rates, hospitalization rates, or mortality rates in relation to Covid-19 unlike the UK where the data concerning ethnic minorities was available from the beginning due to common health care statistics (ibid., p. 6). Even the § 11 of the German Infectious Diseases Protection Act (Infektionsschutzgesetz), which refers to the reportable date in case of infection, records age, gender, and regional/local belonging, does not include ethnicity or migration background. The *RKI* (Robert-Koch-Institute), a federal institute that served as an advisory board to the federal government concerning epidemiological issues during the pandemic, admits to a possible bias in its reception of international Covid-19 research since it favours socio-economic rather than ethnic or socio-cultural exploration and explanation (Wachtler et al./RKI, 2020, pp. 5, 12).

Hence, there is a focus on vulnerability when it comes to detecting and explaining the disproportionate impact of Covid-19 on migrant populations in Germany (Heisig, 2021). In summarizing the state of research, Lewicki (2021) identifies a set of 'risk clusters' based on socio-economic disparities: position in the labour market, overall living conditions, and general health status. The first cluster refers to the higher risk of Covid-19 infection in jobs with little chance of physical distancing, high contact density, and hardly any potential for teleworking. Based on data from health insurance companies it is argued that this applies to those working in care for the elderly but also for other care and health workers, as well as those involved in contact-intensive hospitality and service provision, in general. Someone working in these professions had a five times higher risk of infection than those working in higher education. Migrants, in turn, while they provide 23% of the overall labour force in Germany, are over-represented in the fields of cleaning services with 44%, followed by 36% of those working in care for the elderly, and 34.5% of those employed in postal and other service delivery. Moreover, according to data from labour market research, they tend to be overrepresented in precarious working conditions. For example, 23% of workers with a migration background are employed with temporary contracts in contrast to 10% of the labour force without a migration background (Lewicki, 2021, pp. 3–5; OECD, 2020, p. 9f.; Giesing & Hofbauer Pérez, 2020, p. 43).

The second cluster focuses primarily on the impact of the housing conditions on pandemic resilience. It is argued that people with a migration history find themselves disproportionately in deprived areas, which are characterized by substandard accommodation, overcrowded dwellings, less greenery, and a higher reliance on public transport—all risk factors in times of pandemic. Empirical evidence for this linkage is provided by a study issued by the Berlin Senate from the early Corona period March–October 2020. It indicates a statistical link between high incidence numbers and the high proportion of inhabitants with a migration history, as in such boroughs as Berlin-Kreuzberg (Lewicki, 2021, p. 6f.; Senatsverwaltung Berlin, 2020).

The third cluster suggests an elective affinity between lower socio-economic status and housing conditions with lower health status. Structural disadvantage in the job market and, subsequently, the housing market implies a steady decline in the 'healthy migrant effect' the longer a migration project lasts. Empirical studies, again drawing on data of German health insurance companies, suggest that this lower health status based on socio-economic deprivation has an impact less on the likelihood of getting infected and more on going through a mild or severe dose of Covid-19. For example, being unemployed implied statistically that there was double the risk of being admitted to hospital admission after contracting Covid-19 in contrast to those in regular employment. Evidence suggests that migrants in Germany were hit harder by growing unemployment rates, especially in hotel and service industries (Giesing & Hofbauer Pérez, 2020, p. 43). Furthermore, it became clear that there was a higher risk of Covid-19 comorbidities such as diabetes and ischaemic heart disease among those economically deprived groups, and subsequently the migrant part within these groups (Lewicki, 2021, p. 8f.; OECD, 2020, p. 4).

In addition to these risk factors with a direct socio-economic grounding, Lewicki (2021, p. 9) also mentions that amongst the lower social status groups in German society there was empirical evidence about such risk factors as the lesser inclination to go for check-ups, especially if not free of charge, and the lower likelihood to see a special consultant. However, the OECD (2020, p. 4f.) study labelled these as 'immigrant-specific' risk factors, because they tend to come along with a lack of host-country language proficiency and a subsequent lack of information, which might explain the lower rates of testing for Covid-19 amongst migrant populations. This 'immigrant-specific' perspective is supported by a recent study on health care provision for migrants in the region of Baden-Württemberg, of which Stuttgart is the capital. It argues that it would indeed need a more migrant-specific approach to health care provision if further marginalization amidst scarcer resources is to be avoided (Kluge/Charité, 2023). Generally, Covid-19 has opened up a new playing field for cultural and moral othering. Not by coincidence are Turkish migrants in Germany mentioned amongst those ethnic minorities, who are not just structurally more vulnerable due to pre-existing socio-economic disparities, but who also perceive themselves to be at a greater risk to experiencing CAD (Covid-19-associated discrimination) (Soiné et al., 2021; Dollmann & Kogan, 2021).

The issue of discrimination experience, due to real or felt cultural distance, has proved to be very relevant to assessing vaccination hesitancy amongst residents with a migration background. A study by the above-mentioned RKI institute, based on data gathered between November and December 2021, i.e. during the height of the vaccination campaign, found a significant difference in the vaccination rate amongst the population groups with a migration background (84%) in contrast to those without a migration history (92%). At the same time the study reported that vaccination readiness was higher amongst migrants who were not yet vaccinated migrants (Wulkotte, E. et al./RKI, 2022, pp. 1, 5f.). Next to language barriers the study explains these discrepancies in terms of an experience of discrimination in the field of health care due to accent, appearance, and name (ibid., p. 8). A Munich-based study that focused on Turkish migrants refined these findings (Aktürk et al., 2021). Conducted across six Turkish-speaking GP (general practitioner) surgeries, it initially detected the usual three deterrents as far as Covid-19 vaccination was concerned: complacency (risk perception), convenience (access), and confidence (in the vaccine). However, interestingly enough, this epidemiologically inclined study concluded that there was a need for some more information on the situation of Turkish migrants and their descendants in Germany to understand the broader social dynamics that could explain the distrust of vaccines (ibid., p. 10). Thus, next to conflicting information and conspiracy theories, the study refers to a long-established 'introversion of Turkish immigrants and their rejection of western values' due to 'a lack of successful integration even in the third generation' as a reason for vaccination 'hesitation rather than direct opposition' (ibid., p. 10).

Before we explore this suggestion further through the qualitative research we undertook in Stuttgart, besides the immediate epidemiological impact, two long-term societal consequences of the Covid-19 pandemic need to be mentioned. The first concerns the long-term impact that the pandemic might have had on integration via the education system. It is here that, like in a prism, the aforementioned socio-economic disadvantages of certain segments of Germany's migrant population intersect with the long-term generational prospects of integration.

It is widely assumed for migrant populations in Europe that repeated school closures during the pandemic had a detrimental impact on learning as well as on the integration of immigrant children, especially the younger ones. Handicap factors include initially a lesser degree of access to internet equipment and access to suitable online tutorials, less help by parents busy in pandemic 'frontline' jobs, less access to a quiet place to study, and a potential lack of language proficiency for following online education efficiently (OECD, 2020, pp. 15–19). School lockdowns may have not just had an impact on learning in a narrow sense but might have had a 'hysteresis effect' concerning the so-called second or hidden curriculum. Accordingly, the aftermath of the pandemic may have involved cultural distancing through loss of proficiency in the host-country language, lower aspirations and disengagement from the school system, right up to social isolation, and an overall lack of motivation regarding integration (ibid., p. 18f.).

Early empirical evidence for Germany suggests that the children of refugee-migrants, in particular, went into the school lockdowns with considerable disadvantage. There are also significant differences in learning facilities between school children with and without a migration background, for instance, with regard to access to own PC at home (92% to 85%) or having your own room (88% to 79%). When linked to the assessment of the educational potential of the household, this might in the long terms have considerable consequences. Here it is estimated that 16% of children with migration background live in 'educational poverty' (indicated by the highest educational achievement of their parents) as opposed to 9% amongst those without migration history (Rude, 2020, pp. 46, 49f.).

The second long-term consequence takes us back to where we started this chapter, namely effective membership and societal integration. While the early stages of the pandemic, in particular, worked towards inclusive 'spaces of solidarity', the later stages have re-emphasized hierarchical belonging (Triandafyllidou, 2022). Accordingly, the course of the pandemic has revealed more clearly the ambiguities involved in the integration of migrant populations within a post-migrant society. Although migrants were applauded literally and symbolically as 'frontline essential workers', they were also considered to be a potential 'symbolic threat' due to assumed heteronormative lifestyle (Dollmann & Kogan, 2021), opening up the rift between deserving and underserving members of society. In the balancing act between pandemic risk management and collective solidarity they were included as 'effective members' in participatory action such as quarantine measures but increasing contagion and scarce health resources, such as vaccine, saw them often marginalized in relation to citizens proper. In that respect there might be a 'polarizing effect' (Triandafyllidou, 2022, p. 9) in terms of citizenship and belonging unfolding in the aftermath of the pandemic, because migrants have been simultaneously pulled towards societal membership while at the same time being (more symbolically than effectively) pushed outside the inner circle of those fully belonging.

3.5 The Impact of the Pandemic on Turkish Migrant Integration in Stuttgart

Notions of 'effective membership' and 'deservingness' are indeed the dominant frame in which the pandemic is narrated in our Stuttgart interviews, by both representatives of migrant organizations and 'ordinary' people. Contributing something to society in order to strengthen resilience is a central trope running through the interviews. The middle-aged engineer working for Porsche illustrates the many little extra measures taken by migrant citizens that helped to maintain a sense of normality in society but also gave it a touch of extra civic engagement in a crisis situation:

> *No, thank God not, [no short time work]. A couple of days, maybe a week, but otherwise I was there almost all the time. In my department we had to commission and coordinate the masks, and before that all the tests. You were almost right at the 'front', I have to say. That was also very good for me. I was able to <u>contribute</u> a bit, which was a kind of 'luck' in terms of working together with colleagues. I was lucky to be able to shape a bit of solidarity if you like. [my emphasis]*

In a similar vein the representative of the *DITIB* mosque community recalls the organization of compliance with quarantine rules and lockdown restrictions as a contribution to overcoming a situation of societal crises:

> *Of course, with [distancing] provisions in place, accordingly, were very happy that at least we could temporarily open our mosque, and it wasn't closed down completely. But, um, exactly during the times that there were curfews and so on, we discussed whether we, um, keep our mosque-association temporarily closed, just to make our contribution, um, to the betterment of the society or the pandemic, accordingly, to make our contribution to what will lead to normalisation—this we discussed among one another especially also during Ramadan. [my emphasis]*

As the last interview sequence indicates, these 'civic contributions' were often seen as cultural sacrifice, since social restrictions during the pandemic heavily impacted on the rituals of Turkish culture, starting with Muslim rituals such as Ramadan and the ritual washing of the dead by family members, and ending with such culture-specific modes of sociability as weekly family visits and wedding celebrations with extended kith and kin. Furthermore, in the eyes of many of the people we talked to, this sacrifice was different but very important compared with the more individualized German part of the Covid-19 enforced 'solidarity space'.

In one of our interviews a working class couple near retirement pinpointed this felt difference quite succinctly by referring to two distinct modes of sociability:

> *With Germans, it's simply that they use certain holidays to get together and with us it's simply that we use weekends or certain days off to get together. And that is simply missing. That has simply become rare and I don't think it's going to be like it used to be.*

To really appreciate the social impact of Covid-19 on ordinary Turkish life, we need to delve a bit deeper into the normality of these life-enhancing weekend get-togethers. A middle-aged mother, working as a cashier in a supermarket, reports:

> *Well, it was really hard. We had a seriously ill father, who fortunately actually died at the beginning, so that he didn't live to see it [pandemic]. Then my mother was alone. And then Corona just started. And what we normally do is just that once a week, every Sunday, we always meet up—the whole family,*

really all twenty of us. And we also kept going to see our parents during the week, then later just my mother as well. Uh, and that was just being cancelled then in order to protect her. But she simply didn't get it anymore, right? She just doesn't understand it then why nobody is coming.

The reader might object that this kind of emotional hardship is not completely unfamiliar to non-Turkish members of society with elderly family members. Yet, that is exactly the point. The life-world-related sacrifice that this mother is prepared to make is like the sacrifice that any other member of society for the common good but it is not valued in the same way. She proceeds to link her narrative to the ill-judged and stereotyping media statement by the then Federal Minister of Health about the intensive care units being overburdened by Covid-19 patients from migration backgrounds and, thereby, frames her argument directly within the discourse of 'deservingness' and 'moral citizenship':

Well, I find it [statement made by the Minister of Health] very, very sad. I think that by making our contribution here just like a normal German, and by adapting in the same way, be it in terms of clothing or also with the language, that is—we integrate ourselves really well, 80% of the immigrants. I just think it's a shame that we are always second-class people. So, I think there's a lot, a lot more that needs to be done. Well, we're all—I personally feel more German than Turkish. I think I behave just like any other German here as well. ... That's why I think you just have to differentiate it a bit. [my emphasis]

In their reflections on experiences like this, which occurred when society was in the grip of a pandemic, both everyday and official discourses refer to a framing by 'moral citizenship' and its 'polarization effect'. Everyday discourse has undertones of integration-weariness due to the obvious bifurcation between structural and cultural integration, exemplified in the narrative of the working class couple already introduced:

We are already integrated, but if just we listen to it, integration hasn't quite happened yet. The name already plays a role. If people hear your name, our foreign name, integration is not complete. ... For us personally, I would wish that when I go somewhere, people would say: 'OK, she's not a Turk, she's a normal person here'. But you are still looked at as a blackhead, always as a foreigner. ... They don't say it to your face. We are both German citizens and so, of course, we have equal rights but, let me put it this way, in this society we can't hang our citizenship as a tie on the neck.

However, the same situation was also described with more ideological rigour. Here Covid-19 was never a stand-alone issue but always connected to wider cultural and political cleavages. As the Stuttgart *DITIB* representative explains with the aforementioned statement by the Minister of Health in mind:

> *That is, of course, the discriminating attitude hostile to Islam that was, um, expressed by this person. So, what I've been saying all along was, society is becoming more and more polarised, um, against Muslims, hostility to Islam, islamophobia, group-related misanthropy, those are the big issues that are currently interesting us in our society. And exactly this fire we must not fuel more with firewood by carrying messages into society of the kind that migrants are more afflicted by this disease.*

Because these narratives placed coping with Covid-19 within the general frame of belonging and moral citizenship, we can now take a closer look at two more concrete issues raised by the literature in the previous section: the supposed vaccination hesitancy and the suggested tendency towards introversion by the Turkish community. With regard to vaccination hesitancy, our interviews suggest that the motivation to be vaccinated was shaped by an individual's social position, just as in the wider society. Indeed, one could be tempted to speak of a 'mainstreaming' of vaccination behaviour. The representative of the 'German-Turkish Forum' remarks with a degree of irony:

> *I actually found it quite telling that I, when I looked at, how do you say? corona critics, corona deniers and vaccination critics and so on—[their] comments on social media—repeatedly there were Turkish or other non-German-sounding names involved very prominently. Um, so in a certain way there was also an integration happening here [chuckles].*

The range of views about vaccination that we encountered covered the whole spectrum from routine acceptance to informed hesitancy and opposition. The supermarket cashier referred to earlier on saw the vaccination programme as part and parcel of routine living in Germany: 'And yes, we just got vaccinated blindfold. We live in Germany and I think that, well, is part of it.' The working class couple near retirement felt both encouraged and pressurized by their peers and the social environment: 'The bad thing about it was that people around you always made the rush. We are already and you are not [vaccinated yet].' The facility manager working for the

Stuttgart city council with a general (not just Covid-19 related) interest in alternative medicine needed a bit longer to ponder, only to be eventually 'nudged' by his employer: 'I am actually more in favour of natural medicine, so yes, in the beginning I was against it. But now this opportunity has arisen for city employees, to get the vaccination, and I will definitely take advantage of that.' We also detected evidence of 'hesitation' close to opposition' as mentioned in the previous section of this chapter (Aktürk et al., 2021, p. 10). The person that illustrates this position best is a female student, who is also active in a youth organization attached to the *DITIB* mosque community in Stuttgart. This group, she reports, contributed to vaccination education but she goes on to say:

> *I'm actually one of the late vaccinators. I got vaccinated very late; when I realised that it was no longer possible [to go without]. ... Yes, of course, I do think it is a question of solidarity with others but you should also accept when some people say: 'No. I'll continue to wear my mask.' I also know people who are still not vaccinated because they said: 'I have a home office job, why should I vaccinate myself? I don't go shopping. I order or I usually send my partner shopping or other things.' Yes to solidarity, yes. But having a vaccination injected into your body is another matter of solidarity. To what extent is it ethically justifiable to be put under pressure?*

This could be read as a reflexive understanding of solidarity, where someone refuses to be blindfolded and conform to mechanically imposed rules. They provide solidarity in a differentiated and context-sensitive manner where mutual support is grounded in the changing modes of interdependence between individuals and groups, following Durkheim's famous distinction between mechanical and organic solidarity.

That this layered understanding of solidarity should find a crucial marker in the interlocutor's body should not come as a surprise. Drawing on Paul Gilroy's approach towards the body as 'a cultural locus of resistance' (Schiffauer 2004, pp. 349, 359), it can be argued that the use of the body as a symbolic marker of difference is especially prevalent within versions of Islam in Europe that actively claim a collective right to be different rather than acting as an invisible migrant who is required to see Muslim culture as a personal stigma.

Coming to the second issue, in the previous interview sequence we can detect an intense process of self-reflective repositioning to family, group, and society triggered by Covid-19 and its epidemiological-cum-social consequences at the personal level. However, the direction of this repositioning seems to be more complex than the 'introversion' and 'distancing from Western values' mentioned by the literature (Aktürk et al., 2021, p. 10). At the institutional level of the mosque communities organized by *DITIB* there is a sense of concern about losing the well-kept balance of a 'unique diasporic autonomy' (Öcal & Gökarıksel, 2022, p. 152), which holds at bay both interference by the Turkish state through the Directorate of Religious Affairs that sends and pays the imams in Germany's *DITIB* mosques and the expectation of further assimilation by the German state.

The cooperation with the local state and public policy actors during Covid-19, as emblematically embodied by the joint venture test and vaccination centres attached to *DITIB* mosques, has furthered the pragmatic shift from religious geo-political concerns to 'on the ground realities' (ibid., p. 154). At the same time, however, this has been combined with the downshifting of social life around the mosques, since 'pastoral care', which is a core element of *DITIB* mosque associations (Tezcan, 2008), has moved from the religious and cultural sphere to the realm of state administration.

Some people might see this change as leading to too close an incorporation within local state structures and making the *DITIB* mosques appear like 'outposts of the state in civil society' in times of crisis (Schönwälder, 2020, p. 4). The Stuttgart *DITIB* representative expresses this concern as follows:

> *Accordingly, the daily prayers, religious rituals, and so forth, we have a lot of social activities here, pastoral activities and also cultural activities, that we could no longer, um, organise in presence here. … At the same time, we built up contacts here at the beginning of this month, that is, at the beginning of May, where together with them [local authorities] we then, um, with whom we collaborated and built up a test centre, a test tent in front of our mosque. So far, there has been a brisk demand, and, um, these, well, official tests, they [are] not the self [administered] tests, but rather they are administered under observation. They are also valid at retail and at hairdressers etc., they also have their validity. And we then also thought: 'Why, if we already have a test centre now, we can also set up a vaccination centre'. And we then directly, um, transformed or expanded it in the sense that we also have a vaccination centre, temporary. … But the spiritual, certainly—we have spent two Ramadan, um, months with, the pandemic. So, the spiritual, the communal has suffered a lot. And, um, I'm in hope that, as soon as the pandemic is completely gone, um …, of course we have a fear, that maybe rather fewer will be convening in the community. [my emphasis]*

This fear is by no means unfounded. It ties in with changes at the everyday or life-world level in the Turkish milieu in Stuttgart that point to a more cautious and reflective engagement with extended family and co-ethnics. What was initially an unwelcome and state-imposed restriction of community life due to Covid-19 might turn out to be a useful means for rediscovering community on more individualized terms.

Interestingly, we found this trope present across the spectrum of our interviewees, from the active *DITIB* mosque community member to the Alevi cultural Muslim, from the supermarket cashier to the Porsche master craftsman. The working class couple nearing retirement, who observed Alevi beliefs, describe this development as follows:

> *I also have to say that I'm glad that we have the little restrictions now, so with the whole visit all on it. It was just too much for me before. But you couldn't say no, because it was customary law. And now we've got used to saying: 'Ok, maybe we could have a bit more but we don't want to overdo it. It's just right now. It will be too much if it's really every weekend now.' My husband is still of the attitude: 'Come. We'll call someone. We'll go somewhere.' I'd rather say: 'Come. Let's sit down comfortably at home instead.' It's somehow been accepted that it's more comfortable when you don't have to work so hard over the weekend. It's already becoming a habit that you have the attitude that you shouldn't do it so much. At weddings or something it's like that, thank God it's not as much as it used to be. Four hundred, five hundred people met at these weddings, celebrated together, but it doesn't necessarily have to be. So, it's not the wish: 'Oh, I just miss that'. No, it's a bit reduced and I like that, I think. Or I keep saying it to my husband: 'Could it be that we're getting older, that we're doing a retreat?' But it could also be the effect of the fact that we're used to it now. I don't know.*

While we still find here the inclination to at least partly explain the desire for more self-controlled and selective engagement with the ethnic community in terms of the wear and tear of getting older, the student member of the *DITIB* youth organization leaves no doubt as to the rationalization processes behind this development:

> *You have learned to set yourself limits. Honestly. I had my wedding a month ago now, just under a month ago. I've actually been able to set boundaries because of the pandemic. Even before that, I realised, okay, hey, I don't necessarily have to go there. I don't necessarily have to do it. I can also say, people, I'm sorry. And I also realised that the pandemic has made me more aware of what is important and what is not important. That I can simply break it down and*

say: 'Okay, hey, I want to do this, I don't want to do that. Okay, do I have to go there? Or do I not have to go there?' Well, we can differentiate more now. Because we simply realised because of the pandemic—okay, curfew. Now you have to filter.

The Porsche master craftsman, in turn, is forthright about Covid-19 being used as an excuse of reflexive restructuring of networks in the face of customary law:

That also tailed off during Corona, as did the pastoral care. Yes, how can I put it, to be quite honest. The human being is built in such a way that he avoids this effort. Rather a little less, that's a temptation of sorts. In this respect, there have often been situations where people have been able to talk themselves out of a lot of things under Corona. 'Why they don't do something because they can't do something?' That was such a killer argument. So, a lot of people, in my opinion, were thinking that way.

In order not to give the impression that this development is entirely welcomed by all interlocutors we shall finally refer to the supermarket cashier, who sees these developments more suspiciously:

The family definitely meets up once a week, so there's always—and that is completely gone by now and it's just missed, really. With the restrictions almost gone, it has revitalized slightly, slightly, slightly. It's allowed, but I think at some point you get into a bit of a routine so that you—it has definitely become less. That is, we used to have—we now had the fasting period—it used to be the case during fast that you had visitors or were invited really every day on Friday, Saturday, Sunday. And that's all toned down a bit now. So, everyone has become a bit more cautious and, well. But I think it will come back at some point, or so I hope [laughs].

The account of the repositioning during a societal crisis would not be complete without some discussion about real and imagined embeddedness in transnational space where every German-Turkish milieu is situated to some extent. Somewhat surprisingly, our interlocutors did not talk about disrupted biographies or even divided loyalties. The pandemic seems to have encouraged an even stronger appreciation of what Hannerz (2002, p. 219) has once aptly described as the grounding power of 'everyday territoriality' with its repetitive routine and sometimes boring familiarity, which nevertheless brings a cherished ontological security into everyday life—something obviously very valuable in times of crisis. A 'superior elsewhere' might flash up occasionally but rather as a potential 'escape attempt' from routine, and not as a serious contender for replacing 'home' (Cohen & Taylor, 1992). Indeed, when people talked about the Covid-19 crisis potentially triggering a crisis of belonging, Turkey was usually seen as both a family and a holiday destination. The supermarket cashier, for example, spoke about visiting the family home first and then going on holiday: 'Well, my husband's mum lives in Turkey anyway, and then we always go there first, and then to the beach. She lives near Izmir. And then we just go where it takes us.' For the Porsche master craftsman visiting Turkey involved seeing family and friends rather than taking a holiday: 'When we visit my parents-in-law in Turkey, I don't go on holiday, I am simply with my family, my relatives, my acquaintances'.

The balance between 'home' and 'elsewhere' is expressed most clearly by the student member of the *DITIB* youth organization when she says: 'I don't have to decide between the two but I really do feel at home in Germany. I also say quite frankly that I probably couldn't live so well in Turkey, as I have never really lived there. It's foreign, but still familiar. I like to go there on holiday.' The Stuttgart *DITIB* representative produced the most articulate reflection about people's personal ties to both Germany and Turkey, introducing the important themes of multiple homes and generational change:

> *So, of course there is also a familial connection that we have there. Of course ... Covid-19 has triggered these emotional relations, um, towards our homeland. How are they doing? Whether they are afflicted now, have they got infected, or, um, are they receiving good care? So, naturally, um, questions that interest us just as much as, um, the questions here; only, our scope of action is here, where we live. To put it briefly, um, home is where you, um, first of all, grew up, and secondly, um, where you live. So this is here then, um, the centre of our life, the base where we are, um ... are residing. Of course, our parents came here as guestworkers, but by now we're already in the fourth, you can already say in the fifth generation. Some have very little connection to the country of origin ... and only see it as a holiday destination. But we have to participate here and contribute our involvement here, for this society here.*

The interviews also revealed some proud expressions of regional and local identity: 'I m a Württemberger' (student member of *DITIB* youth organization); 'My children are simply Ur-Stuttgarters, and Swabian' (female supermarket cashier); 'We are Feuerbächler'[1] (working class couple near retirement). Although attachment to the locality rather than to the host country is quite common among migrants (Wessendorf, 2010), there might be something special to Stuttgart after all, as the representative of the German-Turkish Forum suggests:

> *I think this economic prosperity of the Stuttgart region has always been an important magnet, because people have been coming here, but also something that has kept people here. That is, um, when you look at educational successes all the way back to the nineties, um, the share of pupils of Turkish descent in lower secondary schools, or now maybe even middle secondary schools, even special schools, has always been extremely high. But it has never come into play here as much, or didn't have the societal repercussions as maybe in other parts of the country. Um, the Cologne region or also Berlin, um, or the Ruhr region, where a breaking-away of industry and with it the loss of jobs very quickly led to people in fact being left behind socially as well. … we have been spared that so far, fortunately. And because of this the social integration works substantially better perhaps than in other parts of the country, seen nationwide, that is. Um, which of course has left us here in a certain, well, oasis or island of the blissful.*

Whether this is measurable reality or a self-fulfilling prophecy, it does describe well the important role that Stuttgart's economy played during a period of crisis and also what the future might bring.

3.6 Future Integration: A Post-Corona and Post-migration Society

The spirit of 'gear box assembly line integration' is still alive in Stuttgart. Even if post-industrial restructuring has here too shifted a considerable number of jobs from the production line into the service sector (Meier-Braun, 2009), the dream of upward generational social mobility through life-long employment with one of the region's great car manufacturers is still alive, as the Porsche master craftsman illustrates:

> *It is still valid. I have my twenty-fifth anniversary this year, and I have been a master craftsman for 20 years there. I just don't have the engineering degree yet—hopefully, my son will achieve that in a year's time. He is currently studying industrial engineering, and he is also at Porsche AG. Hopefully, he will continue to work there as an engineer when he gets his first proper job as well.*

[1] Referring to locals living in the Stuttgart borough of Feuerbach.

Even those who have not enjoyed social mobility through the car industry enjoy its symbolic prestige, as the facility manager at the Stuttgart city council, who has endured many years of precarious work, testifies when saying: 'We live in the land of automobiles [laughs]—Baden-Württemberg, and I am also happy about it and I like living here'. Thus, this area was in a very strong position when the Covid-19 crisis struck, both in terms of socio-economic integration and in terms of a binding narrative. However, when asked about what lessons have been learned from the crisis the same person responds:

> *One shouldn't use the pandemic to create divisions among oneself or whatever. You should use the pandemic to learn from it how to get closer together once it's over. Because it is only if you talk to each other that you can somehow reach a common denominator and pursue goals that unite us. Whether it takes a long time or not, at some point it will be like that. If you ignore each other, then that will lead us nowhere, let's put it this way. I think we all can live reasonably together, treat each other with respect.*

Other interlocutors responded in a similar way, always stressing that dialogue and (narrative) social engagement was just as important in the aftermath of the pandemic as its technological and administrative processing. The working class couple, for example, recall the one-sided and stereotyping press and media coverage of the Covid-19 infection rate amongst migrants at the height of the pandemic:

> *What is shown on TV is completely different from what happens in reality. And I think it's a pity that everything is thrown into a pile. Something must be put right here. I have the impression that most Germans don't even have experience with foreigners or contact with foreigners. But you can't change that.*

This was said with an undertone of resignation by two people who have been engaged in workers' council and trade union respectively almost all their working life. One of them also served on Stuttgart's 'foreigners' committee' during the late 1990s but found it all 'a bit artificial'.

The supermarket cashier had a long experience of mutual disengagement where there was less emphasis on cultural stereotyping but strong socio-spatial connotations. Living in Bad Cannstatt, one of the Stuttgart boroughs with a rather high residential concentration of people with Turkish roots, she notes how Covid-19 measures have affected long-term integration prospects:

Well, I think it's, uh, worse [than it used to be], for the reason that, uh, well, with my parents the way I knew it was that they simply had German neighbours and they were also grandpas, grandmas to us and, well, we had a much closer connection. At the moment, there are just so many immigrants here, and also people of Turkish origin, that the Turks have somehow turned inwards, I think. And, uh, they just don't want the contact with the outside world anymore. It didn't use to be like that. But because now—it has all evolved even more in a way that the Turks are really more introspective, as simple as that. And so, the coexistence is lacking a bit. And you can also see that here in this neighbourhood especially. There is just a huge crowd of Turks here and they just keep to themselves, which I think is a shame, simply, because, I think, uh, mixing of different cultural aspects just gives us a lot more instead of now just remaining within the Turkish culture. But it's just more difficult, yes.

The Porsche master craftsman for his part rejects the idea that social division 'due to and with' Covid-19 was working like a force of nature:

Covid is a disease of which we don't really know the origin, I cannot really influence it. But hate, division and enmity can have a great influence too, and they are very perceptible, tangible. Because you can see the social context and you can try to act against that to a certain extent in my society, in my neighbourhood, at my work.

These are remarkable statements because, despite being formulated from rather different positions within post-Covid and post-migration society, they all indicate a deep sensitivity towards the life-world of Stuttgart's Turkish migrant population. Firstly, they claim that the pandemic has amplified the social fragmentation and disparities that were there before crisis and they are likely to continue after the pandemic is 'over'. Secondly, they argue that these social divisions cannot be healed by technocratic measures alone, such as catching-up education programmes for migrant children and a better channelling of information by the state through multiplying languages and channels of information. Instead, a narrative engagement across all layers and fragments of society is needed.

Our interlocutors show an awareness that post-pandemic society intersects with ongoing efforts to actively generate a 'post-migrant society' (Foroutan, 2015)—the concept we introduced in the first section of this chapter. Hence, next to such technical issues as the furthering of migrant careers at all institutional levels of society and the transcultural opening of public institutions and services, a society that understands itself as an immigrant society also needs a narrative that reflects this and has the binding capacity for all 'effective residents' as a concrete utopia to be achieved in one's life-time.

The belief in the need for a narrative engagement in a post-Covid/post-migration society is shared by the institutional representatives of the local state and migrant organizations (see also Chap. 2). The deputy head of a Stuttgart borough council declared at the height of the pandemic rather optimistically:

> *Well, things won't be getting worse. Um, I think that after the pandemic you will definitely engage in the conversation more intensively and then also ask people: 'What did you do during that time? How, uh, did you manage to get through it? Have you lost someone to corona, or are you afflicted by long covid in any way?' Well, I do think that a conversation is going to start. ... And then I think that, uh, afterwards then the whole thing will be revived and then maybe all in all, one will move a little closer towards one another again.*

The Stuttgart *DITIB* representative adds in rather philosophical vein: 'We have to ask ourselves, that is a mutual question, accordingly, how we can do more for our society, how we can advocate this mutual interest in a really peaceful society, more just society?' From the representative of the German-Turkish Forum in Stuttgart we can also get the sense that this is exactly where the organization sees its mission and has already gained some knowhow:

> *Well, we organized something like that already some time ago, transferred the so-called East-German/West-German biography talks here into German-Turkish biography talks. That was really exciting. And today I'm convinced that we actually need more such encounters and exchanges.*

Issues that came up in this discussion about a post-Covid/post-migrant society were reflected in the narratives of our Stuttgart interlocutors. Here is an incomplete selection of the lessons/issues that were raised about future integration policy. The representative of the Stuttgart 'German-Turkish Forum' reminds us that improved pandemic communication is not just about better technical channelling of information, but just as much about detailed cultural sensitivity:

When it comes to the issue of vaccination of the elderly, there is a lot of catching-up to do, and the Turks are still a bit of an exception here. We have already seen this with elderly men and women migrants, not all of whom are in ambulant or stationary care, um, who in part are still being cared for at home by family members, who as a matter of fact were not within reach of the mobile vaccination teams going round at the time. They are still not vaccinated until this day, um, in many groups. ... So from that perspective there is surely a migration-specific particular need which, looking back but now also ahead to the coming weeks and months, um, I envision very specifically, where I think, more needs to be done here.

The Porsche master craftsman brings up a rather technical issue that, nevertheless, is of symbolic significance in terms of everyday belonging:

The position of the Muslim in society has become different. You can see that with us. We as an Islamic community moved [into these premises] 17 years ago. Yet the free opportunity for morning or night prayers is still not given. The Islamic community is only allowed to open at 6 o'clock and after 9 o'clock this mosque has to be closed. This is something that then again, a new mayor, definitely might want to discuss with us at some point.

Although both have German citizenship, the working class couple near retirement in their concern for social justice inevitably bring up the unsolved issue of communal citizenship/communal voting for non-EU migrant residents:

So, in some people's eyes you are still a 'guest worker'—but what kind of status is that? If you are exposed to the same duties, then why should you not have the same rights, at least on the municipal level? People living in Stuttgart should have something to say about the political process in Stuttgart.

Recalling her experience of working on a public service hotline at the beginning of the Covid-19 pandemic the student member of a *DITIB* youth organization is sure that 'you definitely need doctors and civil servants with several languages, bilingualism or trilingualism is worth its weight in gold in such a crisis'.

The Stuttgart *DITIB* representative for his part draws our attention to a topic that is not migrant-specific but universal human:

> *Now after the pandemic, we have a big task ahead of us. The pandemic has affected all of us strongly through solitariness at home all the way to there having been psychological, mental disorders, and in the whole of society, that there were encroachments in the familial situation simply because of the overburdening of the children who were also at home. Various factors that we as religious communities definitely, um, have to work through in the pastoral realm all the way to the supporting realm. That is an immense potential that cannot be handily illustrated, with statistics, and many won't admit it but this is a problem that is heading towards us, and a pretty big one. A big snow that we'll then, um, after the opening, might have to absorb.*

The most future-oriented remarks we leave to the representative of the German-Turkish Forum in Stuttgart:

> *Um, then with this debate about the new 'We' in society, or the open society itself, especially in the 2010s, we of course began to increasingly deal with, well, a generation that does not always orientate itself towards Turkey. By now we talk about young people living here in the third or fourth generation, they are no longer merely 'the Turks' or 'the migrants'; they understand themselves very naturally as Stuttgarters or as Cannstatters or as, um, Zuffenhauseners. And how can that be combined with these general questions of identity, problems of integration that have, um, occurred more intensely in the last few decades [along generational lines], until today? Very strong youth groupings, movements have emerged with Black Lives Matter and, um, other initiatives, Fridays for Future as well, um, where the young people are trying to develop a voice of their own. And, um, this development over the past twenty years has been very swift.*

This, then, leaves the final issue to the deputy head of a Stuttgart borough council, who considers the potential for integration in an increasingly individualized society:

> *Because, um, somehow you get the feeling that they [younger generations] are less interested in the community and society overall. But by and large these are almost all individualists, and, um, only in the area of sport—that is where it still works. And there they have a sense of community, so to speak, and, uh, in play and in competing with each other. But, in other areas, as I said, all of them [are] individualists. And I think to myself, it doesn't matter whether it is indeed, uh, with migration or without a migration background, they are all like that at the moment. And so it's not just the pandemic that is to blame.*

3.7 Concluding Remarks: The Outstanding Bill of Integration Policy

'Post-migrant societies are negotiation societies' in search of a cultural narrative that can frame this ongoing negotiation of 'social positions, access, resources and standards', while—and therein lies a certain paradox—this guiding narrative itself can only be imagined as an open and open-ended discourse (Foroutan, 2015, p. 2). The narrative of 'integration', as prevailing in German society, is rather not this narrative—it is, as aptly described by Foroutan, a 'metanarrative' resembling a worldview or ideology. As such, it reduces complexity and gives rather normative guidance for one's own actions and for judging those of others, all this 'from a superordinate perspective' (ibid., p. 4).

In practice, it has developed as an overarching frame of reference from science and policy right 'down' to the nitty-gritty of everyday life. Nieswand (2021) has described this metanarrative, drawing on his empirical study of Baden-Württemberg's migration/integration policy, as 'integrationism'. 'Integrationism', by its very nature, has to be a system of unpaid deeds. It promises the 'established' that the 'newcomer' will integrate without questioning the existing hierarchical order. It promises the 'newcomers' that they will find their place in the hierarchies of jobs within the societal division of labour, as well as in the various roads to cultural recognition and affectual belonging. The last part of the bill—namely, the promise to 'honour' in the truest meaning of the word advances made in integration and adaptation (ibid., p. 91)—remains largely unpaid. Working in this way, the 'integrationism' studied here in the Stuttgart region cannot close the division between structural and cultural integration that lies on the ground of 'moral citizenship' and 'deservingness'.

This leaves the migrant somewhat irritated and resigned. A pandemic, such as Covid-19, has served as a prism of these lived ambivalences. The concluding narrative by the facility manager working for a Stuttgart borough council, who has become familiar to the reader, vividly illustrates this:

> *I also plan to stay here, that is, well, in Germany. I think it's quite okay here, all these opportunities that you have here, you don't have that elsewhere. If you want [it], a door will always open somewhere. … So, I tag along and I don't feel like [a] foreigner or anything. I almost feel like a German, even though I don't look like one but … [chuckles]. Uh, well, my view is that it's sort of equal [with information and vaccination]. Whether it was in 'villadom' at first, or on the 'block', or somewhere else, well, everyone got a chance. Whether they made*

use of it or not is up to each individual—let's put it like that. So, I haven't [noticed] any big differences there. Everyone was treated equally from what I saw and everyone had the opportunity. And, uh, what they made of it, that's up to the individual. ... And, well, I think everyone has got their come-uppance at some point, let me put it that way. At first it was the elderly, and then it was the grandchildren, and then it was the students, and then it was the migrants. Still, that was a completely new experience and you gained experience from it, to look at it that way, but I stand above that. So, I'm not angry about it. If I got angry with every sentence and every word [that conveys stereotypes or discriminates], I wouldn't have any hair on my head [laughs].

References

Aktürk, Z., Linde, K., Hapfelmeier, A., Kunisch, R., & Schneider, A. (2021). COVID-19 Vaccine Hesitancy in People with Migratory Backgrounds: A Cross-sectional Study Among Turkish- and German-speaking Citizens in Munich. *BMC Infectious Diseases, 21*(1–12), 1214. https://doi.org/10.1186/s12879-021-06940-9

Albrecht, S., & Reschl, R. (2005). 'StadtRegion Stuttgart 2030'—Integration in einer segregierten Stadtregion. In Deutsches Institut für Urbanistik (DIfU) (Hrsg.), *Zukunft von Stadt und Region vol.1: Integration und Ausgrenzung in der Stadtgesellschaft* (pp. 53–86). VS.

Barber, B. R. (2013). *If Mayors Ruled the World: Dysfunctional Nations, Rising Cities*. New Haven: Yale University Press.

Campomori, F., & Caponio, T. (2017). Immigrant Integration Policymaking in Italy: Regional Policies in a Multi-level Governance Perspective. *International Review of Administrative Sciences, 83*(2), 303–321. https://doi.org/10.1177/0020852315611238

Cohen, S., & Taylor, L. (1992/1976). *Escape Attempts: The Theory and Practice of Resistance to Everyday Life*. Routledge.

Diehl, C., & Schieckoff, B. (2021). Integration durch Erwerbsarbeit: Vorausset zugen, Herausforderungen und die Rolle der Kommunen. *Stuttgart: APuZ, 71*(5–6), 33–39.

Dollmann, J., & Kogan, I. (2021). COVID-19–associated Discrimination in Germany. *Research in Social Stratification and Mobility, Nr., 74*(100631), 1–10. https://doi.org/10.1016/j.rssm.2021.100631

Eade, J. (2000). *Placing London: From Imperial Capital to Global City*. Oxford: Berghahn.

Emilsson, H. (2015). A national turn of local integration policy: Multi-level governance dynamics in Denmark and Sweden. *Comparative Migration Studies, 3*(7), 1–16. https://doi.org/10.1186/s40878-015-0008-5

Foroutan, N. (2013). *Identity and (Muslim) Integration in Germany*. Migration Policy Institute (MPI).

Foroutan, N. (2015). Unity in Diversity: Integration in a Post-Migrant Society. In *Focus Migration/Policy Brief 28*. IMIS.

Foroutan, N. (2015a). Ein neues Leitbild für Deutschland. Pluralität als gesellschaftliche Aufgabe für die Zukunft. In: Reschke, A. (Hg.) *Und das ist erst der Anfang. Deutschland und die Flüchtlinge* (pp. 283–293). Rowohlt, S.

Frisoli, P., & Mäding, A. (2019). Muslime in Stuttgart 2017: neue Schätzungen zur Zahl der in Stuttgart lebenden Muslime. *Statistik und Informationsman agement* 9/2019.

Galandini, S., Mulvey, G., & Lessard-Phillips, L. (2019). Stuck between Mainstreaming and Localism: Views on the Practice of Migrant Integration in a Devolved Policy Framework. *Journal of International Migration and Integration, 20*, 685–702. https://doi.org/10.1007/s12134-018-0626-5

Geißler, R. (2004). Einheit-in-Verschiedenheit: die interkulturelle Integration von Migranten—ein humaner Mittelweg zwischen Assimilation und Segregation. *Berliner Journal für Soziologie, 14*(3), 287–298.

Giesing, Y., & Hofbauer Pérez, M. (2020). Wie wirkt sich Covid-19 auf Migration und Integration aus? *Ifo Schnelldienst, 73*(7), 41–46.

Green, S. (2007). Divergent Traditions, Converging Responses: Immigration and Integration Policy in the UK and Germany. *German Politics, 16*(1), 95–115.

Guentner, S., & Stanton, R. (2013). Urban Citizenship Through Democratic Variety—Reflections on the Local Political Participation of Migrants in European Cities. *Open Citizenship: Journal for Citizenship Issues in Europe, 4*(2), 38–53.

Hannerz, U. (1998). *Transnational Connections: Culture, People, Places*. Routledge.

Hannerz, U. (2002). Where We Are and Who We Want to Be. In U. Hedetoft & M. Hjort (Eds.), *The Postnational Self: Belonging and Identity* (pp. 217–232). Univ. of Minnesota Press.

Hanson, C., Luedtke, S., Spicer, N., et al. (2021). National health governance, science and the media: Drivers of COVID-19 responses in Germany, Sweden and the UK in 2020. *BMJ Global Health, 2021*(6), e006691. https://doi.org/10.1136/bmjgh-2021-006691

Heisig, J. P. (2021). Soziale Ungleichheit und gesundheitliches Risiko in der Pandemie. In Bundeszentrale für Politische Bildung (Hg.), *Corona: Pandemie und Krise* (S. 332–344). Bpb.

Hepburn, E., & Zapata-Barrero, R. (2014). Introduction: Immigration Policies in Multilevel States. In E. Hepburn & R. Zapata-Barrero (Eds.), *The Politics of Immigration in Multilevel States: Governance and Political Parties* (pp. 3–18). Palgrave.

Hüttermann, J. (2000). Der avancierende Fremde: Zur Genese von Unsicherheitserfahrungen und Konflikten in einem ethnisch polarisierten und sozialräumlich benachteiligten Stadtteil. *Zeitschrift für Soziologie, 29*(4), 275–293.

Joppke, C. (2004). Ethnic Diversity and the State. *British Journal of Sociology, 55*(3), 451–463.

Kimmelmann, M. (2015, October 6). Stuttgart Struggles to House the Migrants it Embraces. *New York Times* [17.05. 2020].

Kluge, U., Hertner, L., & Schödwell, S. (2023). Wenn sowieso das Zeitfenster eng, die Termine rar sind dann sind das natürlich die Leute, die als erstes hinten runterfallen. In *Abschlussbericht Migration und Gesundheitsversorgung Baden-Württemberg (MiG BaWü)* (pp. 1–55). Charité.

Landeshauptstadt Stuttgart Statistisches Amt. (2020). *Datenkompass Stadtbezirke Stuttgart Ausgabe 2019/2020.* Statistisches Amt.

Lewicki, A. (2018). Race, Islamophobia and the Politics of Citizenship in Post-unification Germany. *Patterns of Prejudice, 52*(5), 496–512. https://doi.org/10.1080/0031322X.2018.1502236

Lewicki, A. (2021). *Aktueller Forschungstand: Sind Menschen mit Migrationshin tergrund stärker von Covid-19 betroffen?* Mediendienst Integration.

Meier-Braun, K.-H. (2009). Zuwanderung seit 30 Jahren als Chance und Bereicherung: die Integrationspolitik der Landeshauptstadt Stuttgart gilt bundesweit als vorbildlich. In: Gesemann, F. & Roth, R. (Hg.), *Lokale Integrationspolitik in der Einwanderungsgesellschaft: Migration und Integration als Herausforderung von Kommunen* (pp. 367–382). VS.

Münkler, H. (2018). Zuwanderung und globale Migration als Herausforderung der Demokratie. *Forschungsjournal Soziale Bewegungen, 31*(1–2), 131–138.

Nieswand, B. (2021). Konturen einer Moralsoziologie der Migrationsgesellschaft. *Zeitschrift für Migrationsforschung/Journal of Migration Research, 1*(1), 39975–39995.

Öcal, D. K., & Gökarıksel, B. (2022). Grounding Religious Geopolitics: The Everyday Counter-geopolitical Practices of Turkish Mosque Communities in Germany. *Geoforum, 129*, 151–160.

OECD. (2020). What is the Impact of the COVID-19 Pandemic on Immigrants and Their Children? [oecd.org/coronavirus]

Rude, B. (2020). Geflüchtete Kinder und Covid-19: Corona als Brennglas vorhandener Problematiken. *Ifo Schnelldienst, 73*(12), 46–57.

Schiffauer, W. (2004). Vom Exil-zum Diaspora-Islam. Muslimische Identitäten in Europa. *Soziale Welt, 55*(4), 347–368.

Schönwälder, K. (2020). Diversity and political practice. *Ethnic and Racial Studies, 43*(11), 1929–1941.

Schönwälder, K., & Söhn, J. (2009). Immigrant Settlement Structures in Germany: General Patterns and Urban Levels of Concentration of Major Groups. *Urban Studies, 46*(7), 1439–1460.

Schönwälder, K., & Triadafilopoulos, T. (2012). A Bridge or Barrier to Incorporation? Germany's 1999 Citizenship Reform in Critical Perspective. *German Politics & Society, 30*(1), 52–70.

Senatsverwaltung Berlin. (2020). Das SARS_CoV-2-Infektionsgeschehen in Berlin—Zusammenhang von Soziodemografie und Wohnumfeld. *Kurz Informiert*, 2, 1–10.

Siedentop, S., & Fina, S. (2012). Eine neue Geographie der Segregation? Entwicklungen der ethnischen und generativen Segregation in der Landeshauptstadt Stuttgart. *Statistik und Informationsmanagement*, 10/2012.

Soiné, H., Kriegel, L., & Dollmann, J. (2021). The Impact of the COVID-19 pandemic on Risk Perceptions: Differences Between Ethnic Groups in Germany. *European Societies, 23*(1), 289–306.

Statistisches Amt LHS. (2014). *Stuttgarter Unternehmer mit Migrationshintergrund: Eine Studie zur Stuttgarter Migrantenökonomie*. Stuttgart.

Tezcan, L. (2008). Governmentality, Pastoral Care and Integration. In A. Al-Hamarneh & J. Thielmann (Eds.), *Islam and Muslims in Germany* (pp. 119–132). Leiden.

Triandafyllidou, A. (2022). Spaces of Solidarity and Spaces of Exception: Migration and Membership during Pandemic Times. In A. Triandafyllidou (Ed.), *Migration and Pandemics* (IMISCOE Research Series) (pp. 3–21). Springer. https://doi.org/10.1007/978-3-030-81210-2_1

van Campenhout, G., & van Houtum, H. (2021). 'I am German when we win, but I am an immigrant when we lose'. Theorising on the Deservedness of Migrants in International Football, Using the Case of Mesut Özil. *Sport in Society, 24*(11), 1924–1940. https://doi.org/10.1080/17430437.2020.1865314

Wachtler, B., Michalski, N., Nowossadeck, E., Diercke, M., Wahrendorf, M., Santos-Hövener, C., Lampert, T., & Hoebel, J. (2020). Sozioökonomische Ungleichheit und COVID-19: eine Übersicht über den internationalen Forschungsstand. *Journal of Health Monitoring, 5* (Special Issue 7): Soziale Ungleichheit und COVID-19, 3–18. RKI.

Wessendorf, S. (2010). Local attachments and Transnational Everyday Lives: Second-Generation Italians in Switzerland. *Global Networks, 10*(3), 365–382.

Wessendorf, S. (2013). Commonplace Diversity and the 'Ethos of Mixing': Perceptions of Difference in a London Neighbourhood. *Identities, 20*(4), 407–422.

Williams, H. (2014). Changing the National Narrative: Evolution in Citizenship and Integration in Germany, 2000–10. *Journal of Contemporary History, 49*(1), 54–74.

Wulkotte, E., Schmid-Küpke, N., Neufeind, J., & Wichmann, O. (2022). *Covid-19-Impfquotenmonitoring in Deutschland als Einwanderungsgesellschaft (COVIMO-Fokuserhebung)*. RKI.

CHAPTER 4

Peruvians in Milan: Subsidiarity the Other Way Round

Marco Caselli

4.1 Peruvians in Milan: An Overview

4.1.1 Migration and Migrants in Italy

For over a century, Italy has been a country of emigration, particularly with more than 12.5 million Italians that left the country in the first 30 years of the twentieth century (seriestoriche.istat.it). After World War II, emigration abroad[1] was accompanied by an intense migratory flow from Southern to Northern Italy, a phenomenon which is still present today. Only since 1988 has the Italian migratory balance become positive, with the number of people entering higher than those leaving.

[1] In the 1950s and 1960s, more than 5.5 million Italians emigrated abroad (seriestoriche.istat.it).

M. Caselli (✉)
Dipartimento di Sociologia, Università Cattolica del Sacro Cuore, Milano, Italy
e-mail: marco.caselli@unicatt.it

M. Caselli et al. (eds.), *Migrants' (Im)mobilities in Three European Urban Contexts*, Europe in a Global Context,
https://doi.org/10.1007/978-3-031-53773-8_4

Symbolically, we could consider August 8, 1991—the day the ship *Vlora* arrived in the port of Bari, loaded with tens of thousands of citizens fleeing Albania—as the moment when Italy begin to perceive itself as a country of arrival for migratory flows, and international migrations began to be considered a social problem, which the country clearly appeared unprepared to face (Zenelaga & Goga, 2011). These initial flows, driven above all by the fall of Communist regimes and the crisis in Yugoslavia, mainly came from the former Eastern bloc and some countries around the Mediterranean (Fondazione ISMU, 2020). Although some provisions were introduced during 1990, it was only in 1998 that the first organic law on immigration was enacted (the 'Turco Napolitano' law). This law was followed by others, together with various extraordinary provisions and periodic amnesties. Overall, Italy still does not seem able to produce a clear vision regarding its policies for managing migratory flows and even less of developing a model of integration. In particular, the management of migratory processes has always been faced with an emergency rationale more closely tied to maintaining security than creating stable, consolidated paths for integration (Fondazione ISMU, 2020, pp. 21–23). This inconstant orientation is also echoed in the mood of national public opinion, whose attitudes towards immigration are among the most ambiguous in Europe. While great openness is detected towards foreign citizens already present in Italy, notable fear is shown towards possible newcomers (Fondazione ISMU, 2020, p. 35). One cannot overlook how this ambivalent attitude is also evident across Europe, with policies oscillating between openness and a closed attitude towards migrants (Zanfrini, 2019, p. 6).

A particular trait of Italian migration policies has been the periodic implementation of amnesty measures for undocumented migrants, guided both by humanitarian reasons and by the important role played by these migrants in Italian society, particularly in the fields of family assistance and agriculture. The main amnesties took place in 2002 and 2006. The most recent was enacted in 2020 (Fondazione ISMU, 2021), at the beginning of the pandemic, and this amnesty will be given some consideration at the end of this chapter.

Starting in 2008, mainly due to the economic crisis, migrants entering for work reasons began to decrease while the entry of refugees and asylum seekers grew in importance. These latter flows then exploded in parallel with the Arab Spring and the Syrian and Libyan crises. These developments have meant that in the collective imagination and in the Italian political debate, immigrants are associated above all with the image of desperate people, refugees, etc., although these constitute a very small part of foreign citizens in Italy. Consequently, the management of the foreign presence is conceived, as already mentioned, in terms of an emergency rationale.

In recent years, the growth of foreigners in Italy has slowed considerably, leading for the first time to a slight decrease in the number of foreign citizens between 2019 and 2020. This slowdown is due to the drastic reduction in entries for economic reasons (while those for family reunification remain),[2] citizens returning to their homeland when they consider their migration experience over, and also the progressive acquisition of Italian citizenship by foreign citizens, who have lived in the country for at least ten years.[3]

As regards territorial distribution, foreign citizens are mainly present in Northern and Central Italy, which have better economic and employment prospects. However, in the southern regions, the massive use of immigrant labour in the agricultural sector, often in conditions of real exploitation, should not be overlooked (Fondazione ISMU ETS, 2023; Zanfrini, 2022).

4.1.2 Milan and Migrations

Milan is the principal town in Lombardy, the Italian region that contributes most to national GDP (polis.lombardia.it). Due to its economic and entrepreneurial dynamism, Milan has been the main pole of attraction for migratory flows since the end of WWII, first from the rest of the country, especially from the southern regions (a phenomenon that still exists), and then from abroad (Pugliese, 2006). At the beginning of the pandemic, Milan had a total population of 1,406,242 people (2020), which makes it the second largest city in Italy. The city's urban area is significantly larger, with over 3.2 million people (demo.istat.it).

Eighteen per cent of Milan's residents come from abroad, almost twice the national average. Nearly 17,000 are from Peru, constituting the fourth largest national group in the city, while other substantial national groups include, in order, those from the Philippines, Egypt, and China, followed

[2] For new stay permits issued in 2019, 56.9% were for family reunification, 6.4% for work reasons, 11.5% for study, 15.6% for asylum, and 9.6% for health and other reasons (dati.istat.it).

[3] From 2012 to 2019, 1,061,737 people acquired Italian citizenship (dati.istat.it).

by Sri Lanka and Romania. It is noteworthy that the national groups most present in the Milan area do not correspond perfectly to those, which are most widespread throughout the national territory: the largest national groups in Italy are, in fact, in order, from Romania, Albania, Morocco, China, and Ukraine (demo.istat.it). Migrants in Milan play a key role in providing essential services to local enterprises and families, for example cleaning, deliveries, and home care, but they are also one of the most dynamic players promoting local economy. In fact, Milan is one of the Italian cities with the largest number of enterprises promoted by immigrants (infocamere.it).

4.1.3 Peruvians in Italy and Milan

There are strong ties between Italy and Peru dating to at least the second half of the nineteenth century, when Peru was a destination of Italian emigration and from some regions in particular (Caselli, 2009, p. 31). These relationships explain why, starting in the 1990s, Italy became the main European destination after Spain for Peruvian migrants (iom.int). From a quantitative point of view, the 91,662 Peruvian citizens legally resident in Italy at the beginning of 2020 were strongly concentrated in a limited number of areas around the country. In fact, approximately one-third resides in the Province of Milan, while another third lives in only three other provinces: Rome, Turin, and Florence.

Peruvians maintain strong ties with their country of origin, as evidenced by the fact that despite representing only the 16th national group in terms of the number of people in Italy, they are in 8th place with regard to the volume of remittances. The unemployment rate of Peruvians in Italy is significantly lower than the average of non-EU citizens. Around 0.1% are employed in agriculture, 13.4% in industry, 13.4% in commerce, and 73.1% in services; more precisely, 59% of employed Peruvians work in the personal services sector.[4]

As already mentioned, the city of Milan alone is home to around 17,000 Peruvians, slightly less than the peak of approximately 21,000 reached between 2012 and 2013. This decline anticipated what was reflected nationally for the overall foreign presence and is due to similar causes: the contraction of migration for economic reasons, repatriation, and obtaining Italian citizenship. In particular, there were just under 5000 Peruvians,

[4] Data refer to the period preceding the pandemic. Source: Ministero del Lavoro e delle Politiche Sociali (2020).

who obtained Italian citizenship from 2003 to 2019 (sisi.comune.milano.it). From a demographic point of view, there is a clear prevalence of females among Peruvians in Milan (57.7%, in line with the figure for the whole of Italy, equal to 57.8%), while just over half (51.7%) are aged between 35 and 59 years. From a territorial point of view, Peruvians are to be found especially in the most popular neighbourhoods, but they also appear to be distributed throughout the municipality without any evident form of ghettoization (see Fig. 4.1).

From the qualitative point of view, one could say that, overall, Peruvian citizens in Milan show a good level of socioeconomic integration, to which the language (Spanish and Italian share a certain similarity) and religion (Caselli, 2015) have certainly contributed. This does not mean, however,

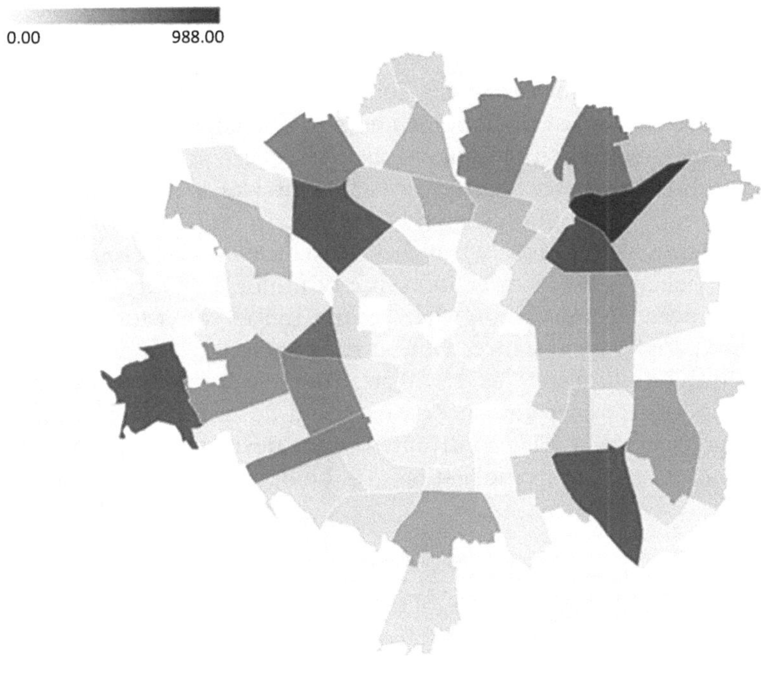

Fig. 4.1 Peruvian residents in Milan (year 2020). (Maps: Marco Caselli—UCSC—Source: Servizio Statistico Comune di Milano—Created with Datawrapper)

that this integration is unproblematic and as we will see below these problems were highlighted by the pandemic. Among the various elements that promoted integration was the ability to enter the job market and the reception and attitude shown by local society towards this national group. Although there was some criticism in the past about the way in which Peruvians used public spaces, since they tended to be particularly noisy and often drank too much, these problems now seem to have subsided. Likewise, in Milan, problems relating to gangs of youths do not seem particularly evident with regard to citizens of Peruvian origin; they have become more significant among other young people, both Italian and immigrants from other countries (Savona et al., 2022; Caselli, 2021). However, the pandemic, in reducing the possibility for large meetings in both public and private space, greatly weakened possible sources of tension with the local community. On the other hand, it also affected an important form of sociability and distinctive social and cultural customs for all Latin American citizens.

With respect to the last point above, it is necessary to mention that identity and the sense of belonging among Peruvian citizens in Milan and in Italy, in general, are multidimensional. They certainly feel Peruvian, but also, in a broader sense, clearly perceive themselves as Latin American. At the same time, many of those, who have lived in Italy for a long time and young people, who arrived when they were little or were even born here, also feel Italian. This identity and sense of multiple affinity may, in some circumstances, be a problem, when feeling Italian is not fully recognized by other people, for instance. During the pandemic, however, as we will see later, this multiplicity was seen as an advantage overall, since it increased the points of reference and those who could be contacted when looking for support and help. This contributed to the development of the 'layered resistance' referred to in the first part of the book.

4.2 The Pandemic in Italy

The first official document published by Italian authorities regarding COVID-19 was the Ministry of Health circular no. 1997, dated January 22, 2020, which officially notified all potentially relevant national and local authorities that the new virus had been identified in China and provided the first indications on conduct if people with related symptoms were discovered in the country. This was followed on January 31, after the virus had been identified in two foreign visitors, by the Council of

Ministers' declaration of the state of emergency for a duration of six months 'as a result of the health risk tied to the insurgence of diseases deriving from transmissible viral agents' (salute.gov.it). On February 23, towns in Lombardy around where the first Italian case of COVID was identified were isolated within a 'red zone', which was then extended to all of Lombardy and some other provinces in Northern Italy on March 8. In the meantime, the closure of schools and universities was decreed on March 4. An initial provision to support workers, businesses, and the national healthcare system was issued on March 17, followed by others on April 8 and May 13. On March 22, a full lockdown was imposed across the entire country, with the closure of all non-essential economic activities, and on March 28, all people coming from abroad were required to declare the reason for their entry, provide a contact phone number, and declare where they would spend a mandatory 14-day quarantine (Cesari & Proietti, 2020; Vese, 2023; Bosa et al., 2022).

Starting on May 4, economic activities began to reopen, although subject to strict health protection measures. Further relaxation of the lockdown and the progressive reopening of all activities, even social and leisure activities, came between May 18 and June 15, although always with the provision of health protection measures. New restrictions were then reactivated starting on October 24 of the same year to confront the so-called second wave of the pandemic (Bosa et al., 2022).

The vaccination campaign began in Italy on December 31, 2020, primarily affecting healthcare workers, and a strategic plan for COVID prevention was adopted on March 12, 2021, with the inclusion of indications and priorities regarding the vaccination programme (epicentro.iss.it). On June 17, 2021, several weeks earlier than what was established on the European level, Italy introduced the EU digital COVID certificate (green pass), issued to people who had tested negative for COVID (valid for 48 or 72 hours depending on the type of test), those who had recovered from COVID (valid six months), or those who were vaccinated. The green pass was mandatory in Italy not only to enter the country but also to access all public places and workplaces. This requirement was then progressively relaxed starting in March 2022, and by the end of the year, vaccination continued to be required only for healthcare workers and those working in hospitals and nursing homes (salute.gov.it). As of June 1, 2022, the green pass was no longer necessary to enter Italy and from January 1, 2023, it was no longer needed when participating in any activities or services (dgc.gov.it).

The effects of the pandemic on foreign citizens present in Italy and those from Peru in particular will be considered in the next section. Here we will discuss the impact of the pandemic on the way in which Italian society perceives immigrants living in the country. This impact has been twofold and ambivalent. On the one hand, the spread of COVID intensified some worrying racist and xenophobic trends that were already present in Italy, leading some to identify citizens of particular nationalities as actual or potential carriers of infection (Riniolo, 2021), a reaction that was also seen in other countries (Haokip, 2021). On the other hand, the pandemic has pushed at least some sectors of society to reflect on the living and employment conditions of many migrants, who worked in conditions bordering on slavery, but nevertheless performed activities that were crucial to the smooth operation of the Italian economy and the endurance of the national welfare system (Zanfrini, 2022). These migrants include, in particular, agricultural workers and those employed in at-home care who, not coincidentally, were the object of an amnesty issued at the start of the pandemic.

One last aspect worth underlining is how, especially in the initial phases of the pandemic, a strong emotional wave developed and a perceptible sense of reciprocal solidarity emerged, not only nationally but also particularly at the local, neighbourhood level. Numerous initiatives came alive more or less spontaneously, from the collection of food for people who needed it most, to concerts and other entertainment organized from balconies, which spread throughout the country on social media. Important demonstrations of solidarity and support were directed, in particular, at those most dedicated to managing and containing the pandemic: law enforcement personnel, and especially healthcare workers, who were offered gifts by some businesses and commercial operators and for whom priority access was reserved at some services and supermarkets. This solidarity was also extended to the numerous Peruvians employed as nurses and healthcare workers as we will see below.

4.3 The Impact of COVID-19 on Peruvians in Milan and Their Response

4.3.1 *The Impact of COVID: Problems and (Tentative) Answers*

For Peruvians living in Milan and in its surroundings, as for all other Italian citizens, the pandemic has had different individual effects, depending on profession, age, health conditions, income, and other personal characteristics. In this respect, among both Italian citizens and immigrants, and in a comparison between these two groups, the pandemic accentuated and further clarified existing differences in terms of income and other material resources, skills, cultural capital, and social and relational capital. In particular, those who already had a stable job, good income and perhaps also some savings, housing that met their personal and family needs, and a solid network of acquaintances and friends in the area before the pandemic managed to face it and its consequences without excessive difficulty or concerns. In contrast, for those who did not possess such resources, the effects of the pandemic were particularly burdensome.

In the specific case of Peruvians, as well as for all foreign citizens, the main discriminating variable was, however, the status of their documents with respect to their residence in the country. It should also be noted that according to the most recent estimates, there are about 11% undocumented Peruvian citizens living in Lombardy.[5]

Therefore, for documented Peruvian citizens the consequences of the pandemic were not significantly different from those experienced by Italian citizens, albeit with a few exceptions. Some lost their jobs, but, in the case of entrepreneurial activities or regular contracts, they were able to benefit from state support and benefits. Others, on the other hand, by virtue of their profession, experienced a period of work overload.

In particular, it is worth highlighting how the pandemic had a particular—and differentiated—effect on some professional areas where the presence of Peruvian citizens (documented and undocumented) was exceptionally high: caregivers and family helpers, delivery workers, cleaners, hotel workers, and healthcare assistants.

With regard to caregivers and family helpers, there were instances—albeit relatively according to the experiences and stories of interviewees—of those who had lost their jobs, either because people were forced to stay home and they no longer needed someone to take care of their children and elderly family members while they were at work, or because people were afraid to let foreigners, and therefore possible carriers of infection, enter their homes. In the case of undocumented workers, this implied a loss in income that could not be compensated with official forms of assistance, given that such aid was reserved for people with a regular job.

[5] Data from ORIM—Osservatorio Regionale per l'Integrazione e la Multietnicità.

A family calls a cleaning lady just for lunch, for a few hours, not for the whole day, there are fewer jobs in this way, people are afraid of contagion on the one hand, and then they have less money on the other, they think: 'I'm at home and why do I need a babysitter all day?' … And immigrant ladies lose their jobs like this. (Leader of a Latin American Catholic group)

More commonly, however, for caregivers and particularly those taking care of elderly people, the pandemic served as an opportunity for more work, although this did not always correspond to an increase in pay and even came near to exploitation and detention. In fact, in many cases, caregivers were prevented from returning to their homes and had to stay at the home of the people they were caring for, or limitations were imposed regarding the activities and movement allowed outside of working hours. This is because the people being cared for were fragile subjects and it was feared that a caregiver leaving and entering the home could be a dangerous vehicle of infection.

Many have lost their jobs, because their employers said to them [home assistants or babysitters]: 'You can't [continue the job] because you'll infect us; so [as an alternative] come and live and work with us and stay with us.' … Those who came to our parish told me: 'I can't be with you and pray because they [employers] are afraid that I will bring contagion to their home'. Then when the situation changed [after the first lockdown] the church reopened and they could not come anyway … because the family where they work did not want that they would go to Mass, and the family where I work asked me too … having done Covid, they … in a certain sense … was more positive … but the family didn't want that I went out. But I wanted to go to Mass! (Leader of a Latin American Catholic group)

In addition, it was shown that in these cases where the caregivers lived 24 hours at the home of the person being cared for, they ended up working many hours beyond what was usual, without being paid a proportionally greater amount. This situation once again highlighted the vulnerable situation of foreign citizens, who are often forced to accept particularly harsh working conditions due to the fear of losing their job and with it both the possibility of economically supporting themselves and their families and the possibility of continuing to reside legally on Italian soil (Zanfrini, 2019, p. 49).

Those who worked in the hotel sector lost their jobs due to the mandatory closure of the facilities where they were employed, but if they were documented, they could benefit from economic support. In contrast, those employed in the cleaning sector, often as small business owners, had a greater workload and also more income. In this respect, one person reported that due to this greater income, it was possible to make up for the money lost by other family members who had perhaps lost an undocumented job.

> *I was lucky though, I was working more. With the cleaning company we sanitized many condos in Milan, we really did a lot of them and often, we always did a double shift, practically every day. … Basically with the overtime and double shift I could make up for the salary that my wife wasn't earning.* (Member of a Latin American Catholic group)

In the course of the interviews, there were many references to Peruvians employed as nurses or public healthcare workers in medical facilities in Milan. These people were on the front lines in the battle against COVID and its effects. They had a very difficult time, both in terms of workload, with often lengthy hours, a greater number of activities to perform, and new procedures to learn, and especially in emotional terms, facing on a daily basis disease, death, and—especially in the initial stages—a sense of powerlessness and inadequacy with respect to the ongoing emergency, which was valid both for Peruvians and for Italians employed in the sector.

> *It was really bad … horrible, there was lots of work to do, loads of work for me, nurses worked very hard and then: loads of suffering and most of all a feeling of total helplessness, it's a feeling that left a mark in me and that shattered me; to be doing a lot but the having the sense of being of little influence. […] I was working normally at the beginning, and then … it blew up. We started with having one person hospitalised and then all of them, the ward was full, then … then all the colleagues, it was truly hard work. We were working very long hours, I can remember those days very well. … I'd get to the hospital in the morning and I wouldn't know what time I'd be finishing. … Almost the whole of 2020 turned out to be like that. No leave, always working, one day after the next. At the beginning I was working in rehabilitation, in the adults ward and in geriatrics, but then … everyone contracted the virus … and then they saw that people were dying so they closed down the ward, and I went to another place, because they were short on nurses. They sent me from one place to the next because there wasn't enough staff. My colleagues were getting sick, and some were in bad conditions. I was always a-symptomatic, I got the virus in November, and I stayed home for 15 days.* (Nurse, member of a Latin American Catholic group)

However, all of this translated into an increase in income through the extraordinary work carried out in a regular context and it also brought a certain prestige and admiration among the community, which we will discuss later in the chapter. Lastly, in the home delivery sector, some small Peruvian entrepreneurs, thanks to the pandemic, were able to significantly develop and consolidate their business.

> *Yes, I, shit, I worked. … I didn't sleep! I wasn't sleeping, do you understand? I also worked on Sundays, in the Covid era. That's where I started working. You know, to me, in quotes, Covid has suited me well. In quotation marks.* (Entrepreneur, leader of a Peruvian association)

As mentioned above, regular Peruvians were able to benefit from the same help and support made available by the state and local authorities to Italian citizens. However, this possibility of economic support and assistance provided to citizens that had a regular job did not mean that even this category of people was without its problems and difficulties. For example, the economic assistance received by employees, who lost their jobs (so-called cassa integrazione), did not fully compensate for the loss in income because this measure did not cover the hours of overtime regularly worked by these employees. This was particularly problematic for those who had a more unstable personal and family situation—for example, those who did not have any savings or had even previously taken on debts and those who lived with people that perhaps lost an undocumented job and, as a result, could not benefit from the same assistance.

Yet, the assumption that migrants were in the same position as Italian citizens with regard to accessing assistance when they lost a regular job was sometimes more hypothetical than real. In practice, some documented Peruvians (but not all) still faced additional difficulties in accessing the aid available due to reduced linguistic competence in Italian. If Peruvians do not have great difficulties in communication in everyday life due to a certain similarity between the Italian and Spanish languages, handling paperwork requires a high level of linguistic skill that not all Peruvians possess.

> *Yes, sometimes I have to go and do the documents, don't I? And there are words there too that I can't understand, and so every now and then I have to be there to ask someone who can help me, because I can't understand [she puts her hands in her hair]. There are words I don't see every day.* (Peruvian girl, working as a cook)

This situation bound up with the pandemic, therefore, accentuated something already noted previously—namely, first-generation Peruvians above all, when they need advice, help, and services, tend to turn above all to Peruvian or Latin American professionals, partly because of these language constraints.

> *But obviously Latinos feel more … how to say? more at ease with another person who speaks their language, and above all who understands their problems, right? And therefore their point of view as a migrant. And then through … through these services, which are still available, I saw that many were able to access them … to [access] some aid, in short.* (Leader of a Peruvian Association)

Moreover, this tendency is facilitated by the good overall level of integration of Peruvians in local society. Many have entered good professional jobs and, therefore, are able to support and provide services to their compatriots. It is also worth mentioning the role played by the Tax Assistance Centres (CAFs). These are private or third-sector companies whose task is precisely to support people in handling paperwork. During the pandemic, Peruvian citizens turned mainly to CAFs that were managed by Peruvian or Latin American citizens. Nevertheless, the fact remains that many of those interviewed declared that they did not encounter specific difficulties during the pandemic.

Even with regard to information retrieval and interpretation, ethnic-based networks of acquaintances and friendship seem to have played an important role amid the informational chaos that Italian citizens also complained about. Some interlocutors mentioned that an important role was played by the numerous Peruvian immigrants employed as nurses and health workers, particularly regarding medical health information.

> *I repeat, we have Peruvians who work in hospitals, right? In hospitals rather than … in that sector there, in short, of health, and therefore they precisely filtered all the information necessary for the community and their families.* (Leader of a Peruvian association)

Like Italian parents, Peruvians with school-age children had to face problems associated with the transition to online teaching in schools, with difficulties made more acute in the case of children with special education needs and large families living in small homes. Yet although these difficulties were certainly relevant, they were not significantly different from those experienced by other Italian children and parents in the same socioeconomic situation (Santagati, 2022; Cordini & De Angelis, 2021). In general, both Italian and immigrant parents found themselves overloaded, having to meet the new needs of their children at a time when an entire series of external support they could normally rely on failed, especially the care and protection provided by schools (Rania et al., 2022).

Forced isolation was particularly hard for the youngest ones, constrained to experience their schooling and social life only online, perhaps within families that did not have a sufficient number of electronic devices or a home large enough to allow each person to have a personal space to guarantee tranquillity and also the privacy necessary to manage their remote interactions. Adolescents in particular, who undoubtedly need a social life of interaction and physical contact, sports and recreational activities, as well as physical space independent from their families for their mental/physical and emotional development, suffered greatly from this situation (Guessoum et al., 2020).

> *I was talking to you about children and young people. I saw a decrease in the relational aspect, with parents and friends, you know. … With parents the tension is normal but during the lockdown you had to stay stuck at home. … The kids have lost enthusiasm, they couldn't go to their friends, they were at home, often they only had one PC, without relationships, without sharing experiences, and without moments of confrontation, then other things started: tensions moved on online chats … strange and stupid things for us but important for them, then you should think to the parents. … They were in a house where there is only one PC … and stop, maybe a phone, then … small houses, we are all closed here. […] The pandemic created an emotional crisis. We followed a good boy—he completely stopped in the pandemic [he was completely disoriented]. He went to hospital, he didn't speak and needed a neuropsychologist—he lost the sense of life. A girl started with emotional crises, she exploded, against her parents. In her view she blamed parents as she lives, it's better for her to die she told us. This hit me too.* (Leader of a Latin American Catholic group)

And this situation had important negative consequences even after the acute phase of the emergency, as the testimonies of school operators demonstrated as well as the sharp increase in requests for psychological support from adolescents (Vicari & Pontillo, 2022). These problems were also experienced intensely by young Italians, but gained particular importance for adolescents of foreign origin, who experienced discomfort even before the pandemic due to their imperfect integration in Italian society and the scholastic environment (Colombo, 2010). This unease was even more intense for adolescents, who arrived in Italy when they were already older, and those who were obliged to migration with their parents, who may have ripped them from the emotional bonds and friendships that they had established in their home countries. Added to this is the fact that prolonged cohabitation imposed by the pandemic in housing, which was not particularly large, often led—and this is also true for Italian citizens—to the emergence or intensification of family tensions, such as those between parents and children, perhaps linked to cases where young people did not choose their migration but experienced it as an imposition.

But the most difficult situation is undoubtedly undocumented Peruvians, especially those who lost their (also under-the-table) jobs due to COVID.

> *With Covid many of them have stayed at home. They tend to earn, work, work, work, often illegally, so without any kind of protection, ok? If you no longer went to work illegally you did not have any form of social protection.* (Officer in the Municipality of Milan)

They were unable to benefit from state aid, but above all, they could not access some basic health services guaranteed to Italian citizens and legal immigrants. Moreover, often due to a lack of dedicated information—which, as some of the interviewees pointed out, the state should have improved during the pandemic—they were unable to access the essential medical services that Italy also guarantees to undocumented migrants without facing the risk that this could lead to deportation (Pasini & Merotta, 2021). However, even before the pandemic it was widely revealed how foreign citizens—and not only undocumented immigrants—were often not fully aware of their rights concerning access to Italian healthcare services (Fondazione ISMU, 2020, p. 32; Merotta, 2011). It is precisely the fear of possible expulsion that led undocumented migrants to minimize their movements—out of fear of possible checks that could be made during the lockdown—and avoided going to the pharmacy or clinics which were also accessible to undocumented residents. Some of the interviewees therefore criticized Italian public institutions, which were judged incapable not only of developing policies but even communication strategies aimed specifically at undocumented migrants. This situation, as underlined above, led to risks not only for the undocumented migrants themselves, but for all of society. If, in fact, a sick undocumented citizen did not access adequate care, which he or she could have taken advantage of, out of fear or a lack of information, that person could become a vehicle of infection for all other citizens.

> *The state … the state didn't even see them [the Peruvians]. I can say I expected this to happen, nothing new, meaning that theoretically as a class they are not so different from others, but in practice they are … because they are a weak class. What the state was especially unable to see, and this is very serious, was the medical implications for all of those who didn't have an Italian health insurance card [undocumented residents], because it's true that if an immigrant goes to a first aid he or she has a right to ad hoc assistance. But if this isn't made clear, people won't know, and this is serious lack of foresight, not just in their regards, but because these people [undocumented Peruvians] leave in close contact with people at risk: they work as baby sitters, cleaners and most of all carers, so they could have acted as powerful vectors for the virus.* (Italian priest in charge for immigrants care)

With regard to the strictly healthcare aspects of the emergency, local authorities noted a problem relating to the issue of vaccinations as soon as they were available. Although these institutions established procedures for even undocumented migrants to access vaccinations, the effectiveness of these procedures was weakened by at least two factors. The first is the one just mentioned: the undocumented residents' lack of information and fear of being intercepted and expelled from the country. The second refers to a lack of specific vaccination incentives for undocumented residents. While Italian or foreign citizens with regular work were in some ways forced to vaccinate themselves in order to continue working, these restrictions were lacking for those—specifically undocumented migrants—who were paid under the table or were even unemployed.

As for the role that public institutions played in managing the pandemic and its consequences, it is worth noting, first, how the Italian welfare system is organized on two levels. As a municipal manager of services for foreigners emphasized, health services are managed regionally, while social assistance is managed by the municipalities. In a situation like the pandemic, where the medical emergency necessitated an increase in assistance, these multiple levels were not conducive to managing various critical situations well.

To try to respond to the emergency situation, the City of Milan set up a dedicated telephone line in the initial days called 'Milano aiuta' [Milan helps]. The purpose was to collect citizens' requests and needs (other than those strictly health/medical related, resulting from the diversification of competencies just mentioned) in order to establish a support network involving civil protection services and various associations and service companies in the area.

> *During the pandemic, right in the very first phase, from the beginning of March 2020, I coordinated the "Milan helps" switchboard so I followed the whole part of … the first phase of emergency. If you remember, it was the one in which we were all really closed at home. […] We were a small group that with the Civil Protection, with the internal volunteers of the municipality or the third sector, we managed this mechanism, a bit of a network with the whole city. So people called us and we hooked them up. The big issues were "I'm here alone", "the shopping", "I have to go to the doctor and I don't know how to go", the carer. […] It was an open switchboard that had very high peaks and who however worked on questions let's say that … that he had created a whole network of … who coordinated all the networks of volunteers in the city. So the person called us "I need the shopping, I need the medicines", and we activated one of the networks to carry the shopping or the medicines, so.* (Officer in the Municipality of Milan)

During the first days of the emergency, the City of Milan also created an email address to collect the availability of individual citizens who were ready to help as volunteers, and it published a call for associations ready to work with the City to support people in situations of need.

Although some of our interviewees stated that the prohibitions and rules to follow were relatively clear during the hardest part of the pandemic, many complained that a certain informational chaos reigned with regard to the available support and services, as well as the subjects to contact and procedures to follow to access such support and services. In particular, it is worth underlining that the difficulties for many Peruvians in getting information about healthcare and bureaucratic issues were noted during the interviews.

However, some suspect that this informational chaos was not tied to the institutions' inability to communicate but rather to the fact that the institutions themselves did not have a clear picture of what should be conveyed. In this respect, one cannot help recalling how the political debate concerning how to implement measures in relation to the pandemic were—in Italy, but also in other countries—rather heated and the strategies for combatting and managing COVID that were, in fact, very different from country to country.

Faced with limited clarity and ambiguous communication—a problem that affected both Italians and immigrants—some of our interlocutors underlined the absence of action and effective communication and listening strategies from Italian institutions aimed specifically at foreigners. In this respect, it is worth recalling, for example, that the above-mentioned telephone line activated by the City of Milan was a service for the entire population and not just immigrants. It can also be added how none of the Peruvian citizens we interviewed mentioned it during the interviews, notwithstanding a specific question about the services and support introduced by local institutions.

If, according to our interlocutors, the local municipal and regional authorities did not implement specific actions aimed at foreigners, it is necessary to underline that they also noted that the immigrants themselves did not expect anything from the authorities.

The suspicion then arises that it is precisely this disillusioned attitude among migrants vis-à-vis the institutions that led them to not interest themselves in and, therefore, not see the actions implemented by the institutions. In practice, a classic self-fulfilling prophecy was triggered: I think the institutions do nothing effective for me, so I do not contact them and, therefore, the actions they eventually do implement wind up being ineffective. In this respect, as noted by the Peruvian manager of a company offering services to foreign citizens whom we interviewed, even before the pandemic, immigrants were not aware of the services that existed and were implemented locally.

> *Because in Italy it is not that there are no services: there are many services, but people don't know it.* (Leader of a Latin American association)

What emerges is a problem that the pandemic certainly contributed to accentuating and making more evident, but which extends beyond the situation of the pandemic itself. This problem relates to communication between institutions and foreigners, as well as the trust that the latter have in institutions, where at least an acceptable level of citizen trust in governing institutions is an essential prerequisite for the overall endurance of the society (Nooteboom, 2007). For example, in terms of trust (and especially the lack of trust) in institutions, one can mention how some immigrants, at least during the first stages of the emergency, were afraid of being taken to hospital in case of an infection, since hospitals were closely tied to the idea of death.

Even before the pandemic, the difficulties in communication and interaction between institutions and foreigners had highlighted the importance of identifying those who could act as mediators between these two entities. In this sense, the very important role that immigrants' associations could play was already clear and it was recognized by institutions, which, even relatively recently, tried to stimulate the birth, formalization, and coordination of associations developed by foreign residents in the area.

Various studies carried out in Milan have highlighted the local presence of a large number of Peruvian associations and this development was explained in the following terms by one of the interviewees, who was president of one of the associations still operating in the area:

> *Let's say it was ... there was a moment in those years, 2005, 2010, right? in which a large part of the community... In my opinion, associations have been an instrument of compensation, right? Because you must consider that many people who came out of Peru were graduates, they were entrepreneurs, they were people who still had a life in Peru ... they were the middle classes. [...] So, arriving here, from the earliest times, finding yourself a doctor, a lawyer, a business administrator, a small entrepreneur, a university professor, a school professor, an engineer... Here we are all equal when we arrive here, everyone. We have to become caregivers, we have to do the cleaning, without removing anything dignified from these jobs, because work dignifies the person. [...] They found themselves doing something that did not give them that personal, professional, human and approach satisfaction. [...] So, associations served in those years ... it was a compensation mechanism, to be able to overcome all the frustrations that people carried around, because they had a baggage of frustration behind them. And therefore, as soon as, in the early days, the immigrant settles down, he/she finds a job, takes a house, reunites the family, then he/she has found his serenity, of family and economic stability. At that point, in the free moment of him/her s/he begins to do something, because we are human beings and we must also find happiness in life, we must do something no matter how simple it is that gratifies us personally. Then associations served to compensate, make people useful and happy. Someone in the field of sport, someone in the field of culture, someone in the field of folklore, someone in... And so many associations were born, which were groups of friends full of good will, to do something that united them.* (Leader of a Latin American Association)

Yet, the potential role of immigrant associations was only realized to a small degree. Immigrant associations were often revealed to be fragile entities with a weak structure and highly reliant on the commitment and passion of a very limited number of people. On the other hand, the institutions perhaps misunderstood the role and nature of immigrant associations, wrongly seeing them as a somewhat official representative of the community in question (Caselli, 2010). There was, therefore, a sort of reciprocal disillusionment between migrant associations and institutions, with the former feeling used by the institutions in a purely instrumental way and the latter not finding the associations to be sufficiently solid partners. However, regarding the capacity and role of immigrant associations, it should be noted how some of them have been adept in developing their activities and, thanks to professional skills acquired over time by some members, were able to provide specific services to both foreign citizens and others.

Amid this framework, the pandemic had a dual impact on the situation of immigrant associations. On the one hand, it slowed if not halted the activities of some of these associations. On the other hand, it also presented new opportunities for action and generated an awareness of what local institutions could do. For local state institutions and the City of Milan, in particular, it was important to rely on the collaboration of immigrant associations or organizations that included non-Italians in their ranks, so that they could more easily overcome the diffidence shown towards institutions by foreign citizens needing some form of assistance.

> *There were some associations that worked with foreign volunteers, in particular one from Corvetto [a neighbourhood in the southern part of Milan] which had a whole network of volunteers who did the shopping. [...] They had foreign volunteers who had made themselves available; that's [very good] because maybe they overcame the barrier of mistrust.* (Officer in the Municipality of Milan)

Yet, this situation once again highlighted weaknesses in the immigrant associations that, during the pandemic, often needed support from other Italian associations and religious organizations in their attempts to help citizens with their difficulties.

Overall, then, mediation between institutions and people needing help during the pandemic—migrants and others—was undertaken by a vast range of entities that during this emergency were often able to work together and with the local institution they aimed to support. These entities consisted of immigrant associations, of course, but also other Italian associations and companies in the service sector, as well as organizations linked to the Catholic Church or other religious bodies. The active role of these associations in managing the pandemic was also shown to be particularly important by virtue of their greater flexibility compared with public institutions, especially because they were less inhibited by bureaucratic formalities. The birth of spontaneous initiatives that were sometimes only scarcely formalized added to this picture. They were promoted by both Italian and foreign citizens and were self-organized. They offered support to people, who had particular needs, by collecting and distributing food or taking shopping to those who could not leave their homes, for example.

Overall, these forms of less-structured assistance, which were often activated or directed through simple word of mouth and promoted and carried out through informal networks—sometimes but not exclusively on an ethnic and/or religious basis—and by civil society organizations and the Catholic Church, or other religious entities, proved to be the most effective in many circumstances for people, who were in situations of greatest need.

In this context, we can and should also quickly refer to the role played by the Catholic Church and other religious entities (the chapter in this book by Molli and Eade is dedicated to the issue and can be referenced for a detailed analysis). Already before the pandemic, the Catholic Church, with its organizations and groups referring to other religious faiths, played an important role in the life of many Peruvian immigrants. The Church served as a point of reference not only for material assistance but also for emotional help for new arrivals, as well as those living in Italy alone without the local support of their families.

> *The [ethnic, Latin American] church is important, it's a pillar. For a newcomer it's fundamental: going to a church means finding people ... the church is a benchmark for all newcomers ... to find and meet those who are already within society. The Church is one of the oldest establishments in the world, it's specialized in helping human beings, in all their aspects. Even at our church [the ethnic church], if someone desperate comes here with their problems and worries, they'll find a priest who'll listen, they'll find prayer and meditation groups that welcome you, and if you're hungry you'll find food here. [...] There's also a Caritas (Internationalis). ... It's important for a lot of families. If you're cold ... you can find clothes and you find contacts. ... This is how it works: I know someone who's looking for a job, I know someone who's looking for a place to sleep ... and the word goes around. The help is given in all directions. ... People are taken care of in this sense.* (Member of a Latin American Catholic group)

Even before the pandemic, religious entities organized solidarity activities that the emergency further stimulated or revitalized where they had dwindled. Among the people we interviewed, those who were most actively involved in religious entities—not just Catholics—emphasized the importance of initiatives seeking to address needs generated by the pandemic.

Some of our interlocutors referred to the role played by the Peruvian Consulate in Milan but it seemed to have a limited reach. Beyond the bureaucratic services commonly performed by consulates, which were mostly provided online during the pandemic, the Peruvian Consulate in Milan also developed assistance networks and acted as a mediator for possible support provided by Italian institutions. However, a few of our interlocutors also mentioned that the mediation provided by Peruvian associations and their managers was sometimes useful in the relationship between immigrants and the Consulate.

Lastly, in relation to the need to find channels and mediators between foreign citizens and local institutions, the role played by CAFs was significant, particularly those managed by immigrants, as mentioned above.

In sum, Peruvian citizens in Milan gained experience from a situation marked by a range of possible assistance and support promoted by different entities, although probably not communicated or recognized with sufficient clarity and perhaps not entirely or adequately coordinated. However, amid this slightly chaotic range, those who needed to, managed to find some form of assistance. As noted below, this situation was very different and decidedly better than what was experienced by their compatriots in Peru, who could not rely on such a wide range of entities ready to provide some form of assistance.

However, it should be noted that many interviewees have somehow and with a certain pride scaled down the impact of COVID on Peruvian citizens in Italy. They have already had to face many complicated situations in their migratory experience, and this, in a certain sense, has forged their character, making them more ready than Italians to face new difficulties, such as those introduced by COVID.

> *Seeing it from the other side, we must say that those who arrive in this country, like me … We have experienced an internal war, terrorism; we have experienced economic difficulties, we have experienced difficult situations… So, a moment like this, it is true, puts us in difficulty, all of us, but we have a capacity to stand up that is perhaps greater because we have already seen it. […] So, one who has lived through this … it's not that we are not afraid, but we have the ability to get back on our feet.* (Leader of a Latin American Association)

Migration involves multiple difficulties. Among Peruvians, this is especially true for those who were among the first to arrive in Italy and Milan, in particular. This involved people who, often educated and with abilities, skills, and perhaps also some economic resources, left Peru to flee not poverty but rather a profound political/social crisis, which posed considerable risks in the present and unsustainable uncertainty for the future. For many Peruvians in Milan today, all of this seems to have led to the development of strong resilience and a capacity to face adversity and rise again afterwards. This capacity is also recognized and underlined by the representatives from institutions and other local entities whom we interviewed.

> *Let's say people with a migrant background have a greater resilience than us.* (Officer in the Municipality of Milan)

> *That being said, I think that they [immigrants] are the ones who reacted in the best way, you'd say resilient, though it's not a word I like very much. Why are they resilient? Because they've been through so much in life that Covid is surely not the worst they've seen. Whereas we Italians were scared, for them trying to survive is a daily job. ... I didn't perceive them as being shocked by Covid and its consequences. [...] So I'd say these two things: they are those who paid the highest price and perhaps also those who reacted in the best way, meaning in the most natural way, because they've been through so much in life that this was certainly not the worse.* (Italian priest in charge for immigrants care)

In this sense, it is worth noting how this resilience drew extensively on current means of communication and social networks. Even before COVID emerged, these resources were used extensively by immigrants, particularly to keep in touch with friends and parents who remained at home or with residents in other parts of Italy or around the world, in addition to sharing information and promoting various types of initiatives, for example, parties, cultural events, or sports tournaments. During the pandemic, they were used in new ways to cope with the restrictions on movement and physical interaction. Many associations were able to continue their activities at least in part by moving them online. Some solidarity and support initiatives for those with the greatest difficulty were also maintained or even started or increased through moving them online. All of this led to the discovery of the potential for remote interaction through these communication tools—a potential that may be used once again after the pandemic is definitively over. For example, the managers of some religious groups showed that moving some moments of reflection and prayer online had allowed them to reach people, who would have been unable to take part had the events been held in person. Caregivers, in particular, come to mind, since they cannot move around freely during the day because they are dedicated to their at-home care activities, but they can, instead, connect online.

In conclusion, it is highlighted how the pandemic—and this is valid not just for immigrants but for society in general—together with its tragic elements also led to positive results and changes that will remain and may lead to appreciable effects on our lives, even after this crisis is definitively over. In an attempt to find a positive aspect even amid this tragedy, the pandemic was nevertheless a moment for collective learning, an aspect that will be addressed specifically in Chap. 5 by Silvia Malacarne.

4.3.2 *Planning the Future*

With reference to how Peruvians in Milan imagine their future, in line with what has already been highlighted in previous research (Caselli, 2011), a rather varied picture emerges. On the one hand, first-generation migrants whose children are well integrated in Italy do not think about returning to Peru; their future is in Italy, alongside their loved ones.

> *I have four children. The eldest is eighteen and the twins are six and then one. … So me … going back to Peru for a visit, why not? But to go back to Peru, to live, and change my life. … My children … [The eldest son] arrived here when he was two, now he is eighteen, so he … doesn't know anything about Peru. He knows what I tell him. Did you get it? The others were born here. I go to Peru to do what? To visit friends. Now … No, I will never go back to Peru. I have a life [here in Milan], I have a family. Now we are opening a new business … [Return to Peru] to do what?* (Entrepreneur, leader of a Peruvian association)

The situation of the youngest Peruvians is different, especially those who have reached high levels of schooling and professional qualification. For some, the prospect of moving to Peru can be tempting because their qualifications could lead to high-level jobs. However, especially for those born in Italy or arriving in the country very young, Peru is a foreign country in many respects, where a considerable effort at integration or re-integration would have to be made after all the effort already made to integrate in Italy. If this is then added to the fact that Peru is a country where political and economic conditions are still considerably unstable, the result is that many members of the younger generation imagine their future in Italy or another country but not Peru. Therefore, with regard to transnational migration, those who have maintained an emotional bond with Peru may continue to cultivate such feelings, perhaps building cooperation or promoting the political and economic development of their home country while continuing to reside in Italy. The picture does not seem to have changed significantly due to the pandemic.

Once again, the situation is different for undocumented Peruvians and those who have not achieved a satisfactory level of socioeconomic integration. As we have seen, the pandemic has often led to a worsening—sometimes even dramatic—of their living conditions and forced them to consider the option of returning to Peru. Yet the pandemic has made this option more difficult due to the blocking of air transport during the first peak of the pandemic and the worsening of social, economic, and health conditions in Peru, which were caused precisely by the pandemic, as many of our interlocutors noted.

Hence, it appears that most Peruvians in Milan see themselves as continuing to stay in Italy, although the first and second generations have different reasons for remaining. Those, who are planning to return to Peru, often believe that they have no alternative. In a nutshell, therefore, it might be said that while remaining in Italy is generally a choice, returning to Peru is sometimes not only a choice but also a necessity. In this sense, the acquisition of Italian citizenship might enable us to distinguish between those, who are making a 'successful' return, that is those who have ended their migration project after acquiring sufficient resources (both economic and skill-based) to enable them to continue their lives in Peru peacefully and with well-being, from those who return due to the failure of their migration project. Returning to Peru with Italian citizenship is, in fact, the preferred option, since it makes the return a non-irreversible choice. Indeed, if the return and reinsertion in Peru turns out to be less satisfying than expected, or if the living conditions and safety there should unexpectedly deteriorate, the possibility of returning to Italy would always remain. The option of 'commuting' between the two countries would also be possible. Again, this complex framework does not seem to have been significantly affected by the pandemic.

The COVID experience does not, therefore, seem to have significantly influenced the ability of Peruvians to imagine their future. In defining their life plans, they have always considered the prospect of having to face unexpected events and difficulties, and COVID is just one of these.

4.4 Final Remarks on the Case of Italy

In Italy after World War II, a deeply rooted political sub-culture inspired by democratic Catholicism combined with the presence of a strong socialist political sub-culture (with the largest Communist Party in Western Europe) encouraged the development and consolidation of a social model that saw the state playing a strong and widespread role in managing, regulating, and supporting social and individual life. This system certainly contributed to spreading a certain level of well-being and security among the Italian population. However, it was also marked by important economic inefficiencies as well as inequities, with some citizens enjoying help and support they did not need while others did not benefit from the system despite being in need.

These inefficiencies and inequities, together with the growing unsustainable national public debt, progressively pushed—and continue to push—towards a revision of the Italian welfare system. In the ensuing debate, the concept of subsidiarity, which became one of the principles recognized by the Italian Constitution in 2001, has carved out space and margins for attention. At the heart of this concept is the idea that the state, and the public sector in general, can and should intervene in managing social life and related problems only where other social actors (such as service-sector entities or even private companies) are unable to satisfy citizens' needs and aspirations.

Given this principle, which has always been difficult to apply in the country (Lodigiani & Pesenti, 2014; Evans & Zimmermann, 2014), the pandemic has brought out what could be called 'subsidiarity the other way round' in relation to the experience of migrants and even others. It was not the state that intervened to overcome the limits and difficulties of the various social actors by supporting their activities where possible, but rather large sectors of civil society—religious organizations, informal networks, and associations of various kinds—that intervened to bridge the gaps in state actions.

Despite some testimonies that emerged from our interviews, this does not mean that the state was absent during the pandemic. It was actually very committed to trying to contain the pandemic and cope with its effects and, not surprisingly, the two most iconic images of the pandemic in Italy are probably those of an exhausted nurse in the national health system and of the Italian army transporting the coffins of pandemic victims out of a small town in Lombardy. All the interviewees also agreed that, during the pandemic, they were happy to be in Italy rather than Peru, given Italian society's better management of the pandemic. Despite its limitations and problems healthcare in Italy is better than in Peru in terms of both accessibility and quality of care, and the impact of the pandemic was much more dramatic in Peru than in Italy.

> *Here in Italy, compared to Peru, the pandemic was very... That is to say that here it is good, let's say that it didn't go like in South America, because in Peru let's say that unfortunately it went bad, because just to go to the hospital cost you what here would be 2000 euro. All the hospitals were full, a lot of people died, really a lot... There were people who maybe didn't have money—that is half of Peruvians is like that—they don't have money, so maybe everyone.* (Peruvian girl, working as a cook)

Nevertheless, the fact remains that despite these great efforts, the Italian state seems to have been rather overwhelmed by the health emergency, especially in the early stages (Moscatelli et al., 2022), due to the lack of adequate preparation for such an event. Consequently, the actions taken by the government were not always consistent (Pellizzoni & Sena, 2021), and the state does not seem to have been very effective in planning specific actions for some people, including immigrants. In response to this difficulty, we have seen the initiatives undertaken by many layers of civil society. So, at the very beginning of the pandemic, Italy introduced amnesties for some types of migrants—family care givers and agricultural workers—but this was not designed in favour of migrants but rather a sector of the national economy (Pasini & Regalia, 2021) that relies on the important contribution by immigrant workers (Zanfrini, 2022). Moreover, the amnesty fits in well with what has always been a general strategy within Italian migration policy, where amnesties for undocumented immigrants have been granted over the years (Ambrosini, 2013), as we mentioned in the first section of this chapter. In the case of the 2020 amnesty, however, it seems to have paradoxically worsened the uncertain condition of many undocumented migrants, since it was substantially blocked through amnesty applications being examined extremely slowly (Morlotti, 2021).

The uncertainty that was consequently generated for many foreigners impacted people's actual situation, creating great emotional unease, which compounded the unease due to job instability and, in common with all Italians and foreigners with regular jobs, the health risks introduced by the pandemic. This uncertainty is also reflected in the ability to plan the future:

[H]ere there is the question of the "amnesty", the regularization for those who are undocumented. The amnesty was born after the first lockdown, but the situation is blocked for the applicants, it is an incredible situation since almost all the requests are still under consideration and those I know in the church are in a strange situation, they are waiting to understand what is going to happen. (Leader of a Latin American Catholic group)

So the periodic recourse to amnesty procedures indicates both the lack of a clear, unambiguous view underlying state migration policy and their partial ineffectiveness. Amnesties are actually extraordinary provisions designed to bridge gaps and adjust limits in ordinary policies. Even before the pandemic, therefore, the management of migration and paths for integration by Italian institutions was problematic—a conclusion that was not only expressed by immigrants but also by scholars and managers of associations and Italian institutions (Fondazione ISMU, 2020, p. 21). While the country could not satisfactorily manage migration at ordinary times, it is not surprising that it did not seem to be able to adequately address it amid an entirely extraordinary situation. The pandemic, in particular, led to overloading institutions since they tried to manage several emergencies at once. The consequence was a failure to pay specific attention to the situation faced by immigrants.

References

Ambrosini, M. (2013). Immigration in Italy: Between Economic Acceptance and Political Rejection. *Journal of International Migration and Integration, 14*(1), 175–194.

Bosa, I., Castelli, A., Castelli, M., Ciani, O., Compagni, A., Galizzi, M. M., Garofano, M., Ghislandi, S., Giannoni, M., Marini, G., & Vainieri, M. (2022). Response to COVID-19: Was Italy (Un)prepared? *Health Economics, Policy and Law, 17*(1), 1–13.

Caselli, M. (2009). *Vite transnazionali? Peruviani e peruviane a Milano.* FrancoAngeli.

Caselli, M. (2010). Integration, Participation, Identity: Immigrant Associations in the Province of Milan. *International Migration, 48*(2), 58–78.

Caselli, M. (2011). Transnational Lives? The Case of Peruvians in Milan. In B. Axford & R. Huggins (Eds.), *Cultures And / Of Globalization.* Cambridge Scholars Publishing.

Caselli, M. (2015). Measuring the Integration of Immigrants: Critical Notes from an Italian Experience. *International Migration, 53*(4), 107–119.

Caselli, M. (a cura di). (2021). *Viaggi, esperienze, ritorni. La migrazione da El Salvador all'Italia*. FrancoAngeli.
Cesari, M., & Proietti, M. (2020). COVID-19 in Italy: Ageism and Decision Making in a Pandemic. *JAMDA, 21*(5), 576–577.
Colombo, E. (a cura di). (2010). *Figli di migranti in Italia. Identificazioni, relazioni, pratiche*. UTET.
Cordini, M., & De Angelis, G. (2021). Families Between Care, Education and Work: The Effects of the Pandemic on Educational Inequalities in Italy and Milan. *European Journal of Education, 56*(4), 578–594.
Evans, M., & Zimmermann, A. (2014). *Global Perspective on Subsidiarity*. Springer.
Fondazione ISMU. (2020). *Venticinquesimo Rapporto sulle migrazioni 2019*. FrancoAngeli.
Fondazione ISMU. (2021). *Ventiseiesimo Rapporto sulle migrazioni 2020*. FrancoAngeli.
Fondazione ISMU ETS. (2023). *Ventottesimo Rapporto sulle migrazioni 2022*. FrancoAngeli.
Guessoum, S. B., Lachal, J., Radjack, R., Carretier, E., Minassian, S., Benoit, L., & Moro, M. R. (2020). Adolescent Psychiatric Disorders During the COVID-19 Pandemic and Lockdown. *Psychiatry Research, 291*, 1–6.
Haokip, T. (2021). From 'Chinky' to 'Coronavirus': Racism against Northeast Indians during the Covid-19 Pandemic. *Asian Ethnicity, 22*(2), 353–373.
Lodigiani, R., & Pesenti, L. (2014). Public Resources Retrenchment and Social Welfare Innovation in Italy: Welfare Cultures and the Subsidiarity Principle in Times of Crisis. *Journal of Contemporary European Studies, 22*(2), 157–170.
Merotta, V. (2011). Welfare e politiche regionali: chi decide che cosa. In N. Pasini (a cura di), *Confini irregolari. Cittadinanza sanitaria in prospettiva comparata e multilivello*. FrancoAngeli.
Ministero del Lavoro e delle Politiche Sociali. (2020). *La comunità peruviana in Italia. Rapporto annuale sulla presenza dei migranti 2019*. ANPAL Servizi.
Morlotti, S. (2021). *Emersione dei rapporti di lavoro: ritardi e ostacoli di una procedura "a rischio"*. Paper ISMU, giugno.
Moscatelli, M., Carrà, E., & Ferrari, C. (2022). Government Support, Active Participation of Families and Optimistic Vision of the Future During the COVID-19 Emergency: Results of a Longitudinal Research Study. *Italian Sociological Review, 12*(6S), 231–247.
Nooteboom, B. (2007). Social Capital, Institutions and Trust. *Review of Social Economy, 65*(1), 29–53.
Pasini, N., & Merotta, V. (2021). Health. In V. Cesareo (Ed.), *The Twenty-sixth Italian Report on Migrations 2020*. Milano.
Pasini, N., & Regalia, M. (2021). The Politics of Immigration in 2020: Regularization and Regional Elections. In V. Cesareo (Ed.), *The Twenty-sixth Italian Report on Migrations 2020* (pp. 99–112). Milano.

Pellizzoni, L., & Sena, B. (2021). Preparedness as Governmentality. Probing the Italian Management of the Covid-19 Emergency. *Sociologica, 15*(3), 61–83.

Pugliese, E. (2006). *L'Italia tra migrazioni internazionali e migrazioni interne.* Il Mulino.

Rania, N., Coppola, I., Lagomarsino, F., & Parisi, R. (2022). Family Well-being during the COVID-19 Lockdown in Italy: Gender Differences and Solidarity Networks of Care. *Child & Family Social Work, 27*, 1–10.

Riniolo, V. (2021). Razzismo e discriminazione ai tempi della pandemia. In Fondazione ISMU (Ed.), *Ventiseiesimo Rapporto sulle migrazioni 2020.* FrancoAngeli.

Santagati, M. (2022). School Closure and Learning Experience in Italy. Giving Voice to Students, Families, and Teachers during the Covid-19 Pandemic. *Rassegna Italiana di Sociologia, 63*(1), 91–117.

Savona, E., Dugato, M., & Villa, E. (2022). *Le Gang Giovanili in Italia*, Transcrime Research in Brief, Serie Italia n. 3.

Vese, D. (2023). Managing the Pandemic: The Italian Strategy for Fighting COVID-19 and the Challenge of Sharing Administrative Powers. *European Journal of Risk Regulation, 14*, 113–140.

Vicari, S., & Pontillo, M. (2022). *Gli adolescenti e il Covid-19. L'impatto della pandemia sul benessere mentale dei ragazzi.* Edizioni LSWR.

Zanfrini, L. (2019). *The Challenge of Migration in a Janus-Faced Europe.* Springer.

Zanfrini, L. (2022). From Slaves to Key Workers? How the Covid-19 Pandemic Questions the Sustainability of the Italian Model of Migrants' Integration. *Rassegna Italiana di Sociologia, 63*(1), 35–62.

Zenelaga, B., & Goga, A. (2011). Reconstructing Self-Identity: The Image of Albanian as 'The Other'. *Journal of Educational and Social Research, 11*(2), 140–153.

PART II

Towards a Sociological Understanding of Layered Resilience

CHAPTER 5

Migrant Mediators as Promoters of Social Cohesion During the Pandemic: An Analysis of the Mutual Learning Process

Silvia Malacarne

5.1 Introduction

The research illustrated in this volume seeks to understand how three minority communities reacted to the COVID-19 pandemic by bringing their own social, cultural and institutional resources into play. This chapter will focus on how some of the migrant mediators we interviewed sought to promote mutual learning in everyday life, contributing thereby to social cohesion.

That the spread of the virus has caused a global crisis with very little precedent is clear for all to see but what has been often overlooked are the positive processes initiated by the pandemic. The health emergency severely tested political, economic and health institutions at a global level.

S. Malacarne (✉)
Dipartimento di Sociologia, Università Cattolica del Sacro Cuore, Milano, Italy
e-mail: silvia.malacarne@unicatt.it

M. Caselli et al. (eds.), *Migrants' (Im)mobilities in Three European Urban Contexts*, Europe in a Global Context,
https://doi.org/10.1007/978-3-031-53773-8_5

In their attempt to find effective solutions to contain and mitigate the crisis, these institutions frequently developed inadequate initiatives in the attempt to reduce the level of uncertainty and vulnerability generated by the spread of the virus (Paul, 2020). In some cases, the crisis has even unmasked 'like a flash' what in 'quiet times' could be forgotten and overlooked (Waltz, 1979, p. 152), such as the inequalities of political and economic power, the lack of institutional effectiveness and legitimacy and the weakness of political collaboration (Colombo & Magri, 2021; De Hann, 2020). Solnit (2009), however, argues that the response to a disaster often involves the 'triumph' of collective action from below, since this action complements or makes up for the failures of public authorities (Mould et al., 2022). It can generate forms of social solidarity that create a common consciousness, a sense of collective responsibility and promote the well-being of society in general. Above all, this kind of action can serve the needs of those who are living in more disadvantaged conditions (Mishra & Rath, 2020).

In this chapter we will illustrate the forms of mutual aid, exchange and mutual learning that emerged spontaneously through informal support networks or as part of initiatives promoted by civil society organizations during the health emergency—reciprocity processes that truly contributed to social cohesion threatened by the crisis and made it possible, as Springer (2020) argues, to survive the pandemic catastrophe.

Keeping in mind the framework outlined above, the chapter will focus on the key role played during the health emergency by a specific category of migrants—migrant mediators. These have a strong sense of belonging to their country of origin but are also firmly embedded in the social fabric of their receiving country, since they know how to access information and communicate in the host language, and mostly hold positions of responsibility at the social, cultural and political level in the host society. Hence, after a brief discussion of the impact that the pandemic has had in general on migrants and minorities, and a summary description of how the concept of mutual learning can be defined with respect to the relationship between migrants and non-migrants, minorities and majorities, the contribution to social cohesion by migrant mediators during the crisis in the three cities will be explored.

5.2 The Ambivalent Effects of the Pandemic on Migrants and Minorities

The onset of the health emergency, caused by the sudden spread of the Coronavirus on a global scale, has affected, albeit in different ways, all countries of the world: from the more wealthy Western countries to poorer countries in the Global South. Some authors contend that the pandemic has encouraged global homogeneity not only in terms of lifestyle but also in ideas and interests (Mishra & Rath, 2020), due to the imposition of restrictive measures established more or less jointly by political leaders, the implementation of globally shared preventative practices and a mutual sense of fighting a universal enemy—COVID-19. This contention reflects perhaps the early stages of the crisis, which involved the first lockdown when people felt united by a common and inexorable destiny and encouraged feelings of solidarity and empathy towards the whole of humanity in danger—a kind of actualization of the Latin *metus hostilis*.

As the emergency progressed, however, the effects of the pandemic became increasingly clear and complex: not only did millions of people lose their lives to the virus but just as many experienced long and traumatic hospitalizations. Furthermore, long-established structural problems came to light, which had never seriously been addressed by those in power (Colombo & Magri, 2021). In particular, socio-economic inequalities emerged (Mishra, 2021) between those who had sufficient resources to easily access medical care, observe the preventative measures or could afford to work safely, perhaps from their homes, and those who had to continue working in order to survive. The latter were confronted by high risks of contagion, inhumane contracts or exploitation without any form of social protection. In addition, the pandemic clearly highlighted two other types of inequality that often overlap: gender inequalities and inequalities linked to ethnicity or nationality. Women and migrants/minorities have turned out to be among the most vulnerable groups during the crisis, as they are highly exposed to health risks in the workplace or as victims of marginalization and social exclusion (De Haan, 2020).

With regard to the impact that the pandemic has had on migrants and minorities, the situation is rather ambivalent globally and the evidence collected in London, Milan and Stuttgart during our study confirms this ambivalence. On the one hand, the health crisis seems to have accentuated the vulnerability of certain categories of migrants/minorities, whose living conditions have made containing the virus extremely arduous. Various forms of stigmatization emerged (De Hann, 2020) as migrants/minorities became easy scapegoats of public opinion (OECD, 2020). Undocumented migrants often had difficulty in accessing salient public health information due to language or cultural barriers (Nezafat Maldonato et al., 2020; O'Reilly-de Brún et al., 2016) or were reluctant to seek health care for fear of exposing themselves publicly and thus risking expulsion from the host country (see Chap. 4). Temporary or seasonal workers who, even before the pandemic, were forced to sign merciless labour contracts, were obliged to live in overcrowded housing, with limited access to medical care and without being able to rely on any social security support. The pandemic has made these kinds of conditions even more severe and risky for the health not only of migrants but of society as a whole (Paul, 2020).

Yet, our study clearly highlighted the indispensable role played by migrant/minority mediators during the health emergency. These mediators have provided support not only to their countries of origin through remittances or exchanging information and experiences through their transnational networks but they have performed the crucial functions of dialogue and mediation within the countries where they have settled, enabling better communication between migrants and non-migrants and thus a more effective pursuit of common challenges. They were engaged on the front line in health care activities, whether at hospital or with private individuals, in home delivery or public and domestic cleaning services, in public transport or in dedicated assembly-line jobs in industries—all occupations that exposed them to a high risk of COVID-19 infection and transmission, while allowing other people (mostly natives) to work safely from home (see Chap. 1). The group of migrant mediators also included those who, by playing a leadership or coordinating role within ethnic associations, institutions and religious organizations, supported those in need during the course of the crisis, both inside and outside their own community.

Based on what has been proposed so far, it can be guessed how the pandemic's impact on migrants has been closely linked to the status of the migrants themselves, to the condition of regularity or irregularity in the receiving societies, the presence or absence of citizenship status and the degree of integration within the country to which they have migrated, which was often demonstrated by a publicly recognized engagement with roles of social and civic responsibility, and, finally, to the capacity for communication, confrontation and dialogue between migrants and the various social actors operating in the country where they have settled. One thing is certain: as some authors have argued, modern, advanced Western systems would not have been as resilient during the pandemic without the assurance of uninterrupted contributions from their migrants (Paul, 2020).

5.3 Mutual Learning in the Scientific Literature: A Look at Migrant Studies

The concept of mutual learning has been deployed in a number of disciplines. For example, in organizational studies, it is associated with the reciprocal exchange between a more experienced member of an organization and a newcomer. Although they perform different roles that place them in an asymmetrical relationship, they can share mutually beneficial resources and thus learn from each other in an equal manner (Kram & Isabella, 1985; Stockkamp & Godshalk, 2022). Moreover, in the context of transdisciplinary research, as Scholz (2000) notes, mutual learning plays a key role thanks to the theoretical and practical dialogue between researchers and non-academic actors (Lang et al., 2012; Pettibone et al., 2018; Vilsmaier et al., 2015). An exchange process can be generated that stimulates the creation of new knowledge, but also the integration of already existing knowledge. Therefore, it is a valuable form of collaboration, capable of triggering mutual learning processes among all parties involved in the research, and leading each to benefit from cooperating with the other, ultimately seeing their own starting knowledge expanded (Häberli et al., 2001). The mutual learning theme also finds its place in the field of participatory action-research projects, where researchers and potential research beneficiaries work closely together to find common solutions to jointly identified problems (Ngoma, 2022; Beks et al., 2022; Hazard et al., 2017). This approach supports the process of mutual learning between participants through collective reflection, since it involves them in co-design work where each can bring their own resources to bear, teaching and learning from each other (Högfeldt et al., 2019).

The international relations field is another sector where the concept of mutual learning has been deployed. Here, mutual learning is associated with dialogue and integration between Western principles, which have traditionally been shaped by international relations theory, and non-Western conceptual categories, which seek to enhance specific local experiences in order to support the creation of truly global knowledge (Eun, 2018). These de-Westernization and democratization processes of scientific knowledge, to which the perspective of mutual learning can contribute, have also proved to be fundamentally important for international development cooperation. This cooperation is today strongly oriented—at least theoretically—towards promoting equal forms of exchange between countries in the Global North and South through the realization of increasingly inclusive partnerships, designed to pursue human and sustainable development without leaving anyone behind (Caselli et al., 2021; Chaturvedi et al., 2020; OECD, 2018).

With regard particularly to international development cooperation, mutual learning can be described as a process of sharing resources that are heterogeneous in nature and value (theoretical knowledge, technical skills, experience, practices, cultural systems, development models) in a context of asymmetrical relationships. However, mutual learning aspires to achieve an equal exchange between the actors involved so that they can teach and, at the same time, learn from each other. The theme of mutual learning in the context of development cooperation is based, therefore, on the three related aspects: (1) reciprocity, (2) learning, processes that take place within (3) a system of asymmetrical relationships, such as those between donor-beneficiary or helper-helped (Isabekova, 2021). Given the deep connection between the development cooperation sector, particularly in its co-development component, and the area of transnational migration (Malacarne, 2021), these three aspects will be used as a point of reference for the analysis of the interviews carried out in the research we have undertaken in Milan, London and Stuttgart.

With regard, more specifically, to the relationship between mutual learning and migration, Goodkind (2006) has shown how mutual learning can be considered a process that seeks to improve the well-being of migrants. In other words, it is a strategy designed to overcome the hierarchical logic of aid and minimize the power differentials between migrants and those who offer to support them. One of the most valid approaches towards promoting and protecting migrant well-being—not only physical and psychological, but also economic, social and cultural—through mutual learning is to develop programmes based on social contact between people from different backgrounds and cultures, such as between a particular migrant community and the country of settlement. In such a condition of exchange, an authentic sharing of knowledge, skills, experiences, lifestyles, cultural codes can take place, which enhances the strengths of each person's belonging and avoids marginalization (Philips et al., 2014; Goodkind, 2006). Continuous contact between aid providers and aid recipients is essential (Isabekova, 2021), where the sharing of common practices and cross-cultural dialogue not only allows an in-depth understanding to develop between the parties and thus a mutual and bidirectional learning process (Constantine & Shankland, 2017), but also helps to dispel false myths and break down stereotypes and prejudices between people from different backgrounds (Philips et al., 2014).

In order to initiate and support processes of this kind, however, it is necessary to go beyond a needs-based model, which assumes the presence of vulnerable individuals with needs that must necessarily be met through a top-down approach by those who, at least apparently, possess more resources. We need to adopt a perspective that places trust in migrants and their capabilities, capable of promoting and supporting the building of equal relationships with non-migrant communities, according to the logic of mutual learning (Malacarne, 2021).

Another particularly significant study focusing on the relationship between migrants and mutual learning was conducted by Van Ewijk (2012, 2016) and concerns five transnational municipal partnerships established between the Dutch government and the local governments of Morocco and Turkey, respectively, with the aim of delving into the role played by migrants in these partnerships. The main reason for Dutch institutions deciding to initiate these partnerships was the belief that fostering cooperation between migrants' countries of origin and destination in the Netherlands would also promote their better integration into Dutch society (Van Ewijk, 2012). Indeed, the research results showed a strengthening of ties between Moroccan and Turkish local governments and Dutch municipalities, mainly thanks to the generation of mutual learning forms related to cultural exchange and the interaction of differences. After all, as Johnson and Wilson (2009, p. 26) note, it is difference, not commonality, that is the source of learning and new knowledge. Van Ewijk's study also highlighted the crucial role of migrants within these types of partnerships and emphasized their function as facilitators of mutual learning between the different actors involved. In the areas of cooperation between these countries of origin and destination countries, migrants have performed multiple functions: they have established new projects, fostered communication by mediating between language varieties and coordinated exchange field visits. Migrants brought an awareness of the cultural specificities of the countries of origin (in this case, Morocco and Turkey), technical skills developed in the countries of origin and translation skills in the local languages that proved to be an indispensable resource for the effectiveness of exchanges between partners (Van Ewijk, 2016, p. 388).

5.4 Migrant Mediators as Facilitators of Mutual Learning During the Pandemic in London, Milan and Stuttgart

Some scholarly contributions have shown how the onset of the health emergency represented not only a moment of great despair and uncertainty for the whole of humanity, but also turned out be a genuine chance for change in favour of global society, which, suddenly confronted with the pandemic challenge, naturally gave collective space to feelings of generosity and altruism and practices of solidarity and mutual aid. These feelings were deeply at odds with the dominant capitalist and neoliberal logic, focused on selfish interests and individual profit maximization (Mould et al., 2022; Springer, 2020). Although the deep 'human' connection between individuals and their sense of communion has weakened since the emergency, it is undeniable that in some cases the health crisis proved to be an opportunity to rediscover values and experiment with practices aimed at the good of others. For instance, some authors emphasize how the dissemination of COVID-19 has triggered virtuous processes of help and solidarity or activated multiple forms of mutual exchange and learning among people—social cooperation strategies that are vital in resisting the crisis and collectively overcoming it (Mishra & Rath, 2020; Mould et al., 2022).

Some of our research data shows how intercultural exchange and dialogue, mutual learning and solidarity also occurred among Bangladeshi, Peruvian and Turkish residents in London, Milan and Stuttgart, respectively. Therefore, the next section will briefly examine our study's most significant findings starting with the concept of mutual learning and its main components (reciprocity, learning and relations between the Global North and South) and the key role of migrant mediators in activating collective processes of exchange and mutual learning.

5.5 Forms of Reciprocity

The interviews reveal traces of reciprocity that mostly take the form of mutual aid with charitable purposes, a concept also highlighted by Mould et al. (2022) to identify the philanthropic and altruistic *modus operandi* frequently adopted by charities during the pandemic. Ethnic associations, religious communities, civil society organizations or informal groups worked hard to meet the basic needs of people in distress during the health emergency, such as the lack of food, medicines and economic resources. They also filled the need for spiritual, emotional and psychological support caused not only by the isolation or social distancing imposed by governments but also by the climate of fear generated by the rapid spread of the virus.

> *The community has come together a lot to support vulnerable people, especially around sort of the food banks and the people who are suffering, so neighbours or community groups getting together, supporting each other supporting people in their locality in the streets and the areas, we were going out delivering food to people … So I think the community as a whole has come together to support people. (London, Bangladeshi political activist)*
>
> *We … do counselling for people, this is from a psychological and emotional point of view, and this in a period like the pandemic, and even afterwards, has been crucial, people need to talk, to share. It's human … Then we also give help—let's say, practical help. If someone has some needs they ask. (Milan, Head of a Peruvian Evangelical Church)*
>
> *So, that it was especially during the fasting period, during the breaking of the fast, that the mosque communities distributed these food parcels in the neighbourhood. But now in the general area, well, precisely because of this very strong retreat into the private sphere, you didn't really notice very much of it. (Stuttgart, Managing Director of German-Turkish Forum Stuttgart)*

Just as what happens at the theoretical level in the mutual learning perspective, our data suggests that reciprocity has involved an exchange of heterogeneous resources between multiple actors, with different origins and backgrounds, each with specific roles and peculiarities. During the pandemic, formal and informal groups often worked to promote activities that brought migrants and non-migrants together in order to build a dynamic network through which access to and dissemination of useful services and information to the most marginalized and vulnerable was ensured. Digital platforms were set up, sometimes involving professionals and experts, and opportunities were organized for dialogue and discussion on health, socio-economic, political and educational issues related to the different contexts of residence. People had the opportunity to ask questions, clarify doubts or share reflections.

Some of our interlocutors believed that the exchange processes that emerged and were encouraged during the pandemic helped to strengthen the relationship between people from different cultural backgrounds and thus promoted the consolidation of social cohesion.

We experienced during the pandemic situations where we helped each other in different ways and each one of us got help and were supported and empathized by somebody from a different community, so a lot of white people had service, were supported, cared for by Black and Asian and whatever and everyone is helping everyone else, the impact of the love and the support and the hard work that everybody did to help each other, so I think there is going to be an impact on promoting community cohesion. (London, Bangladeshi member of the Stepney Community Trust and Brick Lane Circle Organization)

In the building where I lived you could see that there was exchange. To tell you the truth, it was something new, the building was, in fact, in a particular situation, because on the first floors all foreigners, four out of five flat, on the upper floors lived Italians, so those upstairs complained about too much noise from those below, before it was like that but then [during the pandemic] seeing the basket with charity things was a nice signal. (Milan, Peruvian member of a Catholic-inspired Italian organization)

So the things that we normally do in presence in our associations, we moved to online platforms as good as possible. Apart from that, we also held info events regularly on the corona, restrictions or changes accordingly. And also, of course, on vaccines, we cooperated with our networks, with doctors, where we informed, one the hand, in German, and also in Turkish, about the vaccine in general, right up to side effects, whether or not, which vaccine … (Stuttgart, Dialogue representative of DITIB Württemberg)

5.6 Forms of Learning

Smith and Elliott (2007) divide the relationship between learning and crisis into three different forms. The first—'learning for crisis'—constitutes a process where those involved develop responsive and reactive skills towards the critical event. The second—'learning as crisis'—identifies a kind of crisis that calls into question established beliefs or basic assumptions about a particular organization, thus generating 'turbulence' with respect to the *status quo*, and encouraging new learning. Finally, the third—'learning from crisis'—recognizes the possibility of learning from first-hand experience or from the experiences of others, in order to establish more effective precautionary norms or resilience strategies for dealing with possible future crises.

All three forms of learning emerge from our data. First of all, with respect to 'learning for crisis', the response by public institutions and civil society as well as individuals' response to the challenges posed by the spread of the virus developed quickly and took diverse forms. At the macro level, governments imposed restrictive and containment measures, while forms of solidarity and support were generated by actors operating at the meso level of society while some citizens offered individual help to more vulnerable relatives or neighbours. With regard to 'learning from crisis', some respondents believed that experience of dealing with the pandemic could help people to learn new strategies for dealing with a future emergency.

I don't have high hopes that something will change when everything goes back to normal again, but maybe you can somehow learn more from it for the next natural disaster. (Stuttgart, Managing Director of the German-Turkish Forum in Stuttgart)

Particularly relevant are the forms of 'learning as crisis' that are associated here with the introduction of new practices, which were initially somewhat destabilizing, but which proved to be increasingly indispensable, as the months went by, for carrying out various daily activities, both at an individual and a collective level. A clear example was the innovative use of technology, especially digital platforms, as indispensable tools to keep people in touch and open a channel of communication that was essential for dealing with the crisis. Migrants and non-migrants intensively used smartphones or personal computers to communicate with their family members, who very often lived in far-away countries. Numerous associations or religious communities also acquired skills in using these devices to enable their members and faithful to participate virtually in community activities or religious rites.

But the pandemic taught us how we can use the internet and technology to do some of the things that we used to do, so now, one of the impacts of the pandemic is that you can combine online meetings with physical meetings because everyone is familiar with online meeting, you know Zoom and Teams and whatever so, in the future you won't have to have ten meetings in a venue, so you save the venue cost that way and also you don't overburden people so you can have less physical meeting. (London, Bangladeshi member of Stepney Community Trust and Brick Lane Circle organization)

When this happened we were done with face-to-face meetings. But we were the first to do meetings via the Internet. We were already doing many activities on Skype, then we used other programmes (Zoom). From this point of view we were already familiar with distance worship. (Milan, Head of a Peruvian Evangelical Church)

A doctor of Bangladeshi heritage, who was born and raised in the London borough of Tower Hamlets and worked in the British National Health Service, tells how he created a WhatsApp group to raise awareness and pass on reliable information to other Bangladeshis in the area. Over time, this initiative proved to be a vibrant platform for exchange and learning concerning various issues—first and foremost, the importance of undergoing the COVID-19 vaccination.

> *I just made a WhatsApp group, went on various forums and shared the link saying: 'Hey, this is a Tower Hamlets Covid forum and this was way before the vaccine' and so started building up an open safe space for people to come and talk about people's fears or pressures that they have. [...] When the vaccine was deemed safe by MHRA, then it started becoming a vaccine confidence platform and trying to encourage people to learn the right information, debunk any misinformation and then help them spread positive messages throughout the community. (London, NHS Bangladeshi doctor)*

Our interlocutors frequently linked learning practices developed during the pandemic to the use of technological tools that were rarely considered in the past. Our data confirms the holistic and multidimensional nature of this learning, as is typical of the mutual learning perspective. This kind of learning activates different human capacities, not only cognitive and rational ones but also social and emotional ones; it is intimately connected to the possibility of learning from experience and the social relationships that develop, albeit sometimes virtually, in a given social context.

5.7 Forms of Mutual Learning

The forms of reciprocity and learning that emerged during the pandemic and were reflected in the data collected in London, Milan and Stuttgart can be included in the conceptual framework of mutual learning, since they are inherent to relational dynamics that confront migrants and non-migrants. In fact, as seen above, one of the constituent elements of the mutual learning construct introduced here is the presence of a context in which actors from the Global North and South have the opportunity to interact and thus experience mutual learning practices.

As we will see, the interviews show how these reciprocity and learning processes were driven by a specific category of migrants (migrant mediators), who were engaged with the host society through important professional roles or leadership or coordination functions within ethnic or religious associations. They played key roles during the health emergency both in support of those from their country of origin, with whom they nurtured a deep sense of belonging, and towards the host society, with which they actively operated and maintained a lively dialogue with political institutions.

5.7.1 In London

Firstly, in the London borough of Tower Hamlets, local community and political activists including the so-called Covid Champions seem to perform the role of mutual learning facilitators very well. They are members of the Bangladeshi community (doctors, leaders of local organizations, young community workers, business people, mosque worshippers), who got involved by helping those most in need during the health emergency, both inside and outside their own community. They distributed masks, provided useful information about the vaccine and its potential, assisted lonely or sick elderly people and so on.

> *We've figured out that there's a need for me here to tell my community or even people on my estate what the new direction is and what to do and not do... so I think that idea about helping each other ... and wanting to know just what's happening and spread the message locally has become quite huge. [...] The Covid Champions were going out and speaking to people and giving away masks and PPE and giving out information about what the vaccine is about so people get to understand what is really happening. (Bangladeshi borough councillor)*

Bangladeshis, who wanted to help, were assisted by their local political representatives, in a process that fostered mutual exchange and learning practices:

> *I know somebody, [who] wanted to help when we were attacked by the pandemic and so he would contact the local councillor here and ask him who needs help, who should I go and support and the councillor would say: 'There's this guy in this block or somebody who needs help or who needs some shopping to be done'. So he would then go and do that on behalf of that person but being signposted by a councillor in the first place. (Bangladeshi member of the Swadhinata Trust, a local heritage organisation)*

The Bangladeshi doctor's testimony, already mentioned above, was particularly significant here. He describes himself as a bridge builder between fellow Bangladeshis and others. On the one hand, he engaged in a lively and prolonged dialogue with the government and local political institutions with the aim of acquainting them with the particular difficulties that Bangladeshis were facing both before and during the pandemic. He drew on his personal experience to ensure that these institutions implemented policy actions appropriate to the context and real needs of local Bangladeshis. On the other hand, he remained anchored to his community by serving it as a doctor. He explained, for example, to both community leaders and ordinary people the meaning of some preventative measures as well as the importance of adopting a particular lifestyle and taking specific medicines in case people contracted the virus.

This doctor drew on two key skills to facilitate mutual learning practices between migrants and non-migrants. Firstly, he could communicate in both English and Bengali and this skill, coupled with his authoritative role as an NHS doctor, gave him a lot of credibility and enabled him to gain the trust of both fellow Bangladeshis and his NHS colleagues. Secondly, he drew on his experience of growing up in the locality as well as his spirit of service to the social welfare of society as a whole:

> *I felt like a middleman … because a lot of the people that I care about or that I want to serve are my friends and family and people that I have personal connections with … And so when I go to these meetings with government and policy makers and people who make the big decisions, it's a personal battle because I can see it from their point of view … when people talk about mistrust or when people talk about overcrowding. I grew up in a two bed house, a two bed flat in Stepney Green with eleven people staying there. No policymaker can explain overcrowding to me because they've read it in a book or they've read it in a paper, I've lived it. […] I'm able to tell my parents what their medications mean or how to change their lifestyle or how to navigate the healthcare system and I can do the same for my siblings and I can do the same for my community … When the vaccine was … recommended by MHRA [Medicines and Healthcare products Regulatory Agency] and was being rolled out, I was able to talk to my community leaders. I did a Q & A with the Imam from the East London Mosque on BBC Asian Network in Bangla talking to people about the vaccine … I did loads of media work—all in Bangla—just to help people understand that … So it wasn't just an individual's benefit. And I think people are starting to realise that, … you know? When we talk about social mobility*

> *and we talk about widening participation, ... we have to appreciate the community's benefit and the benefits to society as well ... I truly think that's the way forward for the lessons learned in terms of the ethnic engagements. (Bangladeshi NHS doctor)*

5.7.2 *In Milan*

Those who can best be described as migrant mediators and thus facilitators of mutual learning seem to be the Peruvian migrants, who were engaged on the front line at Milan's hospitals as nurses or socio-medical workers, even during the most arduous stages of contagion. They collaborated closely with Italian doctors, working almost non-stop at an exhausting pace, caring indiscriminately for both Italian and migrant patients. They proved, therefore, an indispensable resource in preventing the collapse of the Italian health system, so severely tested during the health emergency by a constant shortage of personnel.

> *It was really bad. It was a period with a lot of work for me, the nurses worked a lot and then, so much suffering and especially so much helplessness. The feeling of helplessness is something that marked me and affected me—doing a lot but feeling that I had little impact. ... I was working normally at the beginning and then it all started. We went from one in-patient to everyone, the ward was full, then all the colleagues, it was very tiring. Very long shifts. I also remember those days well. I would arrive in the morning and didn't know when I would finish. Almost all of 2020 was like that. No rest, always working, one day after the other. ... At the beginning I worked in rehabilitation, adult ward and geriatrics but then everybody got infected. And then they saw that people were dying and they closed the ward and I went to another location. There were no nurses—they made me go around because there was a shortage of staff. ... [And in the Peruvian community] many people got sick, but I would say few serious ones. But when we knew somebody got sick everybody moved, all of us mobilized: the food, the groceries and the medicines, we helped each other so much. Those, who stayed at home, those who couldn't go out, those who had no money, those who had problems—everyone, each other. (Member of a Latin American community)*

The pandemic certainly highlighted the key role of these Peruvian migrants, who unhesitatingly engaged in health care operations within Milan's hospitals and private homes to support the elderly and sick, mostly Italians. These migrants were able to act as bridge-builders between the

Latin American migrant communities and the wider society within the area, because their professional role helped them to quickly transmit useful information to deal with emergencies, explain the meaning of certain preventive practices and provide material aid and spiritual support, inside and outside their communities of origin.

> *So many Peruvian women, but also men … I saw the situation of women, who had the opportunity to become nurses rather than OSS … They were employed full time, during the pandemic. And so, in that case, it was just the opposite situation—that they were in such demand, that they were always busy, that maybe they even did things that were not their responsibility, because there was a lack of staff. And so they became important and here is the contribution of the foreigner, the migrant. … On their side, maybe they already knew how to move, with their families, or at least they advised because they were inside this … no?—inside the hospitals. And so a lot of things they saw, a lot of things maybe they said. And so on that side maybe there was less difficulty … They simply had, so to speak, maybe the good fortune to be there and therefore to be personally informed or to experience certain situations at first hand. So they were doing word of mouth, with the community. (Milano, President of an Italo-Peruvian association)*

5.7.3 In Stuttgart

The case of Stuttgart centres around the exchange between the Turkish migrant community and the wider German population where the facilitators of mutual learning involved two particular organizations rather than particular individuals. The German-Turkish Forum and the Turkish-Islamic Union of Religious Affairs brought together associations that belonged to different mosques within the area. The data we collected shows that the intermediary function performed by these organizations was already well defined before the onset of the health emergency. The Managing Director of the German-Turkish Forum in Stuttgart, who was one of those interviewed, pointed out that the Forum was born precisely with the intention of building bridges between the Turkish and German sections of the population. It was not one Turkish migrant association among many, nor was it an umbrella organization for other Turkish associations. It focused on keeping alive the contact and interaction between the Turkish communities in Stuttgart and public institutions or other entities in Germany, in order to foster the production of shared ideas and the construction of joint projects, capable of generating forms of mutual learning for all groups involved.

But, we notice very strongly how important these exchanges are with cultural institutions in Stuttgart, because all of these informal opportunities for exchange have to be created, in part, for mutual ideas to arise. And for this, such encounters are very important. ... We are in probably dozens of working groups on the local level from health planning to the Haus der Kulturen that is to be created, where we are in constant exchange with other local institutions or municipal, offices and agencies. And the exchange is, in fact, very important, because we can achieve something with the projects that we organize and, likewise, with the capacities and resources that we have. (Managing Director of German-Turkish Forum in Stuttgart)

The pandemic highlighted the crucial role of such organizations in encouraging exchange, dialogue and mutual learning between the Turkish population and German society. The already active cooperation between different actors in the area made the synergetic work to cope with the health emergency more agile.

We are living here in a society—we only have one society here, in which we all live together. Whether it be ethnical, cultural, religious, accordingly, plays absolutely no role. We have one society that we live in and which, we here must maintain in a peaceful way and in good cooperation. The stronger the institutional, contacts, the higher the trust, the quicker a cooperation is able to succeed. And when we now have to do job XY together, then the trust is already there—the hurdles are no longer there. This makes the work immensely easier—... that you know directly in a trustful cooperation. It is a team work, nothing else. ... And there you have this trust, that you have a blind trust, roughly that the trust is very big so that you, can work much better and more qualitatively and, faster. (Dialogue representative, DITIB Württemberg)

5.8 Conclusions

This chapter has covered three issues: the emergence of the COVID-19 pandemic, the plight of migrants during the health emergency and the role of migrant mediators as facilitators of mutual learning processes, who helped people to cope with the crisis and also strengthened social cohesion. What is certain is that the pandemic has sent a very clear message to the West, namely, that 'its' migrants represent indispensable resources, without which the advanced systems of the Global North would not have been so resilient (Paul, 2020).

Yet, why are migrant mediators so important in fostering mutual learning practices? They occupy a key position in the receiving society, since they are interstitial figures between two or more countries, cultures and traditions (Marini, 2015) and are, therefore, in a particularly strong position to facilitate the development of mutual learning processes. They draw on their experience of mutuality based on their intermediary, bifocal and active position between the country of settlement and the country of origin. They also draw on their learning, which they have acquired through the process of transition from their country of origin or, for second-generation migrants, from the phase of bidirectional acculturation and adaptation in the destination country (Malacarne, 2021).

By proactively cultivating their dual identity and mediating between their countries of origin and destination, these mediators can both encourage more equal and balanced forms of exchange and support a virtuous circuit that contributes to a more integrated local development (Mezzetti et al., 2009). Therefore, thanks to their overcoming the welfarist approach that perceives actors in the Global North as coadjutors of those from the South, they contribute to a perspective where migrants are seen as actors and promoters of development in the country where they reside and operate. They make in other words an important contribution to intercultural exchange.

Finally, we would like to mention two critical issues that have emerged from the chapter and can contribute to further debate or research. The first concerns the temporary nature of the forms of solidarity, help, exchange and mutual learning that were triggered by the health emergency. These forms gradually waned as the pandemic became increasingly 'normalized', raising the question as to how social cohesion between migrants and non-migrants can be stimulated in 'normal times', without a mutual enemy to fight. This question should become a central issue for both public institutions and those working in civil society organizations at a time when the relationship between foreigners is a daily reality in every society, at least in the Western world.

The second issue concerns irregular migrants. They carry out clandestine work or perform roles, which are not fully recognized by the society in which they reside. They are more exposed to forms of marginalization and social exclusion under ordinary conditions but were even more vulnerable during the health crisis for a number of reasons. Many lost their jobs, had difficulty in receiving information dedicated to emergency management, were unable to access essential health services, sometimes for fear of incurring expulsion practices, and so on. A serious effort should be demanded from governments and public institutions in Western countries to provide them with widespread social protection services, to streamline the bureaucratic paperwork related to the reception system and to promote forms of reintegration based on dialogue between migrants and non-migrants, so that all can become full-fledged actors of mutual learning and thus of social cohesion.

References

Beks, H., Amos, T., Bell, J., Ryan, J., Hayward, J., Brown, A., et al. (2022). Participatory Research with a Rural Aboriginal Community Controlled Health Organisation: Lessons Learned Using the CONSIDER Statement. *Rural and Remote Health, 22*, 1. https://doi.org/10.22605/RRH6740

Caselli, M., Malacarne, S., & Rotondi, C. (2021). Cooperazione Internazionale Allo Sviluppo. *Dizionario di dottrina sociale della Chiesa. Le cose nuove del XXI secolo, 1*, 49–56. https://doi.org/10.26350/dizdott_000006

Chaturvedi, S., Janus, H., Klingebiel, S., Li, X., Mello e Souza, A., Sidiropoulos, E., & Wehrmann, D. (2020). Development Cooperation in the Context of Contested Global Governance. In S. Chaturvedi et al. (Eds.), *The Palgrave Handbook of Development Cooperation for Achieving the 2030 Agenda: Contested Collaboration* (pp. 1–21). Palgrave Macmillan. https://doi.org/10.1007/978-3-030-57938-8_1

Colombo, A., & Magri, P. (Eds.). (2021). *Il mondo al tempo del Covid. L'ora dell'Europa?* Ledizioni LediPublishing.

Constantine, J., & Shankland, A. (2017). From Policy Transfer to Mutual Learning? Political Recognition, Power and Process in the Emerging Landscape of International Development Cooperation. *Novos Estudios Cebrap, 36*, 99–122. https://doi.org/10.25091/s0101-3300201700010005

De Haan, A. (2020). Labour Migrants During the Pandemic: A Comparative Perspective. *The Indian Journal of Labour Economics, 63*, 885–900. https://doi.org/10.1007/s41027-020-00283-w

Eun, Y. (2018). Beyond 'The West/non-West Divide' in IR: How to Ensure Dialogue as Mutual Learning. *The Chinese Journal of International Politics, 11*(4), 435–449. https://doi.org/10.1093/cjip/poy014

Goodkind, J. R. (2006). Promoting Hmong Refugees' Well-Being Through Mutual Learning: Valuing Knowledge, Culture, and Experience. *American Journal of Community Psychology, 37*(1/2), 77–93. https://doi.org/10.1007/s10464-005-9003-6

Häberli, R., Bill, A., Grossenbacher-Mansuy, W., Klein, J., Scholz, R. W., & Welti, M. (2001). Synthesis. In J. Klein, W. Grossenbacher-Mansuy, R. Häberli,

A. Bill, R. W. Scholz, & M. Welti (Eds.), *Transdisciplinarity: Joint Problem Solving among Science, Technology, and Society. An Effective Way for Managing Complexity* (pp. 6–22). Birkhäuser Verlag. https://doi.org/10.1007/978-3-0348-8419-8_2

Hazard, L., Steyaert, P., Martin, G., Couix, N., Navas, M., Duru, M., et al. (2017). Mutual Learning between Researchers and Farmers During Implementation of Scientific Principles for Sustainable Development: The Case of Biodiversity-based Agriculture. *Sustainability Science, 13*(2), 517–530. https://doi.org/10.1007/s11625-017-0440-6

Högfeldt, A., Rosén, A., Mwase, C., Lantz, A., Gumaelius, L., Shayo, E., et al. (2019). Mutual Capacity Building through North-South Collaboration Using Challenge-Driven Education. *Sustainability, 11*(7236), 1–30. https://doi.org/10.3390/su11247236

Isabekova, G. (2021). Mutual Learning on the Local Level: The Swiss Red Cross and the Village Health Committees in the Kyrgyz Republic. *Global Social Policy, 21*(1), 117–137. https://doi.org/10.1177/1468018120950032

Johnson, H., & Wilson, G. (2009). Learning and Mutuality in Municipal Partnership and Beyond: A Focus on Northern Partners. *Habitat International, 33*(2), 210–217. https://doi.org/10.1016/j.habitatint.2008.10.013

Kram, K. E., & Isabella, L. A. (1985). Mentoring Alternatives: The Role of Peer Relationships in Career Development. *Academy of Management Journal, 28*(1), 110–132. https://doi.org/10.2307/256064

Lang, D. J., Wiek, A., Bergmann, M., Stauffacher, M., Martens, P., & Moll, P. (2012). Transdisciplinary Research in Sustainability Science: Practice, Principles, and Challenges. *Sustainability Science, 7*, 25–43. https://doi.org/10.1007/s11625-011-0149-x

Malacarne, S. (2021). Migrazioni transnazionali e cooperazione internazionale allo sviluppo: un dialogo possibile grazie all'esperienza di mutual learning. In S. Acampa, G. Gargiulo, & R. Gatti (Eds.), *Saperi, conoscenze ed esperienze in formazione. Atti della V conferenza nazionale delle dottorande e dei dottorandi in scienze sociali* (pp. 353–360). Libreriauniversitaria.it.

Marini, F. (2015). *Co-sviluppo e integrazione. Le associazioni ghanesi in Italia e nel Regno Unito*. FrancoAngeli, Milano.

Mezzetti, P., Rogantin, F., & Russo, M. (2009). *Associazioni di migranti senegalesi: nuovi attori per lo sviluppo. I bisogni formativi delle associazioni senegalesi in Italia alla luce di alcune esperienze di capacity building europeo a confronto.* Centro Studi di Politica Internazionale. Retrieved May 2023, from https://www.cespi.it/sites/default/files/documenti/wp10_mezzetti.pdf

Mishra, C., & Rath, N. (2020). Social Solidarity during a Pandemic: Through and Beyond Durkheimian Lens. *Social Sciences & Humanities Open, 2*(1), 1–7. https://doi.org/10.1016/j.ssaho.2020.100079

Mishra, D. K. (2021). Migrant Labour during the Pandemic: A Political Economy Perspective. *The Indian Economic Journal, 69*(3), 410–424. https://doi.org/10.1177/00194662211021209

Mould, O., Cole, J., Badger, A., & Brown, P. (2022). Solidarity Not Charity: Learning the Lessons of the COVID-19 Pandemic to Reconceptualise the Radicality of Mutual Aid. *Transactions of the Institute of British Geographers, 47*, 866–879. https://doi.org/10.1111/tran.12553

Nezafat Maldonato, B. M., Collins, J., Blundell, H. J., & Singh, L. (2020). Engaging the Vulnerable: A Rapid Review of Public Health Communication Aimed at Migrants during the COVID-19 Pandemic in Europe. *Journal of Migration and Health, 1*(2), 1–6. https://doi.org/10.1016/j.jmh.2020.100004

Ngoma, C. (2022). Mutual Learning during Post-implementation. A Study of Designing a Maternal and Child Health Application in Rural Tanzania. *Scandinavian Journal of Information Systems, 34*(1), 1–40.

O'Reilly-de Brún, M., de Brún, T., Okonkwo, E., Bonsenge-Bokanga, J. S., De Almeida Silva, M. M., Ogbebor, F., Mierzejewska, A., Nnadi, L., van Weel-Baumgarten, E., van Weel, C., van den Muijsenbergh, M., & MacFarlane, A. (2016). Using Participatory Learning & Action Research to Access and Engage with 'Hard to Reach' Migrants in Primary Healthcare Research. *BMC Healtth Services Research, 16*(25), 1–16. https://doi.org/10.1186/s12913-015-1247-8

OECD. (2018). *Development Co-operation Report 2018: Joining Forces to Leave No One Behind*. OECD Publishing.

OECD. (2020). *What Is the Impact of the COVID-19 Pandemic on Immigrants and Their Children?* Document available online. Retrieved April 2023, from https://www.oecd.org/coronavirus/policy-responses/what-is-the-impact-of-the-covid-19-pandemic-on-immigrants-and-their-children-e7cbb7de/

Paul, R. (2020). Europe's Essential Workers: Migration and Pandemic Politics in Central and Eastern Europe during COVID-19. *European Policy Analysis, 6*(2), 238–263. https://doi.org/10.1002/epa2.1105

Pettibone, L., Blättel-Mink, B., Balázs, B., Giulio, A. D., Göbel, C., Heubach, K., et al. (2018). Transdisciplinary Sustainability Research and Citizen Science: Options for Mutual Learning. *Gaia* (Heidelberg, Germany), *27*(2), 222–225.

Philips, D., Athwal, B., Robinson, D., & Harrison, M. (2014). Towards Intercultural Engagement: Building Shared Visions of Neighbourhood and Community in an Era of New Migration. *Journal of Ethnic and Migration Studies, 40*(1), 42–59. https://doi.org/10.1080/1369183X.2013.782146

Scholz, R. W. (2000). The Mutual Learning Sessions. In J. Klein, W. Grossenbacher-Mansuy, R. Häberli, A. Bill, R. W. Scholz, & M. Welti (Eds.), *Transdisciplinarity: Joint Problem Solving among Science, Technology, and Society. An Effective Way for Managing Complexity* (pp. 117–129). Birkhäuser Verlag. https://doi.org/10.1007/978-3-0348-8419-8_11

Smith, D., & Elliott, D. (2007). Exploring the Barriers to Learning from Crisis. *Management Learning, 38*(5), 1–20. https://doi.org/10.1177/1350507607083205

Solnit, R. (2009). *A Paradise Built in Hell.* Penguin Books.

Springer, S. (2020). Caring Geographies: The COVID-19 Interregnum and a Return to Mutual Aid. *Dialogues in Human Geography, 10*(2), 112–115. https://doi.org/10.1177/2043820620931277

Stockkamp, M., & Godshalk, V. M. (2022). Mutual Learning in Peer Mentoring: Effects on Mentors and Protégés. *Mentoring & Tutoring, 30*(2), 64–183. https://doi.org/10.1080/13611267.2022.2057100

Van Ewijk, E. (2012). Mutual Learning in Dutch-Moroccan and Dutch-Turkish Municipal Partnership. *Window of the Netherlands, 103*(1), 101–109. https://doi.org/10.1111/j.1467-9663.2011.00698.x

Van Ewijk, E. (2016). Engaging Migrants in Translocal Partnership: The Case of Dutch-Moroccan and Dutch-Turkish Municipal Partnership. *Population, Space and Place, 22*, 382–395. https://doi.org/10.1002/psp.1872

Vilsmaier, U., Engbers, M., Luthardt, P., Maas-Deipenbrock, R. M., Wunderlich, S., & Scholz, R. W. (2015). *Case-based* Mutual Learning Sessions: Knowledge Integration and Transfer in Transdisciplinary Processes. *Sustainability Science, 10*(4), 563–580.

Waltz, K. N. (1979). *Theory of International Politics.* Addison-Wesley Publishing Company.

CHAPTER 6

Resisting, Reacting and Reinventing: Exploring the Role of Minority Religious Solidarities in Milan and London During the Pandemic

Samuele Davide Molli and John Eade

6.1 Framing Minority Religions and Their Role(s) at the Time of the Pandemic

When considering the multifaceted relationship between state capacity and the everyday lives of migrant minorities during and after the pandemic, the role of religion is crucial. There are various reasons for studying why and how religion played an important intermediary function during

S. D. Molli
Dipartimento di Scienze Sociali e Politiche, Università degli Studi di Milano, Milano, Italy
e-mail: samuele.molli@unimi.it

J. Eade (✉)
University of Roehampton, London, UK
e-mail: J.Eade@roehampton.ac.uk

M. Caselli et al. (eds.), *Migrants' (Im)mobilities in Three European Urban Contexts*, Europe in a Global Context,
https://doi.org/10.1007/978-3-031-53773-8_6

this crisis, but it is also necessary to consider how this function was shaped by factors which preceded the crisis and reflected different nation-state processes (Eade, 2011).

Over time and with varying intensity, different political orientations and ideologies have informed the ways in which religion operates in the public sphere (Barbalet et al., 2011), where different government strategies, juridical frameworks and policies of regulation operate through both cooperation and conflict. The regulation and monitoring of religion by the state is a key feature of European social history, but it has been increasingly challenged by the development of new religious solidarities as a result of transnational migration. Whether and how these solidarities can reduce or reinforce trust in and compliance with state institutions has become an important question today, especially if we consider that religions are often a significant factor in the lives of minority migrants. The attempt by states to regulate religious pluralism from above has often been challenged from below by new religious solidarities, which are informed by social and cultural influences bound up with transnational migration.

Human beings often turn to religion when faced with unexpected disasters and tragedies. They seek in religious beliefs and practices answers to insecurities, the alleviation of suffering, resistance to stress and hope for the future (Del Re & Naso, 2022). The 'anchoring role' played by religion became a prominent feature after the arrival of the COVID-19 pandemic (Molteni et al., 2021), particularly for many members of the migrant minorities who faced the emergency without being able to draw on the wide range of relational, family, political and economic resources that many native citizens had at their disposal.

As well as providing comfort, which helps to encourage mental and psychological resilience (e.g., Connor, 2012), religious solidarities can support migrant minorities through a complex range of cultural, civic and social benefits (Hirschman, 2004). These solidarities facilitate the creation of transnational continuities that link past and present and permit the exchange of meanings with the homeland (Levitt, 2007), but they also become a source of practical support by developing safe relational networks, welfare projects, civic partnerships and aid campaigns (Ambrosini et al., 2021a, 2021b). The polysemous and polyvalent character that faith usually develops when people migrate explains why many migrants put their trust in religious institutions when they settle in another country (Ambrosini et al., 2022) and, equally, why it is important to explore their role in filtering and mediating the impact of the pandemic.

The health emergency imposed a series of changes and challenges, especially those involving the response to state interventions, such as lockdown regulations and social distancing (Giordan & Palmisano, 2022; Ricucci & Bossi, 2022). These had a deep impact on the *modus operandi* of religious institutions and their relationship with the faithful. Moreover, the duties imposed by the emergency guidelines not only involved religious practice but also symbolic issues (Pace, 2021), i.e., which types of 'goods and values' should be given priority during a crisis. The state asserted its authority by appealing to biomedical and economic arguments (Colombo, 2021) and other perspectives were relegated to second place. The state determined what was 'central and essential' for people during an emergency, while concerns about religious freedom were sidelined. This misalignment needs to be carefully considered when analysing the civic involvement of religious actors and their commitment to reinforcing compliance or reducing trust. This is even more crucial in the case of migrant minorities since they often lack institutional recognition as well as suffer discrimination from public authorities.

The problems generated by the pandemic crisis depend on a complex set of transnational, national and local factors, such as the ethno-religious ties associated with particular religious sites, agreements and/or juridical accords with public institutions, the capacity of both religious leaders and lay people to interpret state regulations and health crisis for others, their willingness to promote civic tasks and develop caring networks. Other factors were involved such as the citizenship and juridical status of congregants as well as their gender and socio-economic composition. The intersection of these different factors meant that the unequal impact of the pandemic took various paths (Bonizzoni & Dotsey, 2021) shaped by differences in legal position (from long-term permits to the condition of irregularity), job situation, family condition and social capital (Maestripieri, 2021; Pastore, 2021).

Hence, while restrictive policies imposed by authorities applied to everyone, such as 'stay at home', the intersection of macro-, meso- and micro-level factors led to different ways of responding and reacting. This chapter seeks to explore this diversity by concentrating on Latin American Catholics, especially of Peruvian origin, in Milan and Bangladeshi Muslims in London. With regard to Milan, we will consider the role of three ethnic churches, while in London we will focus on those associated with two mosques in particular as well as a local funeral director.

Adopting a local-level perspective provides the opportunity to compare how macro-processes have been reinterpreted and readjusted by members of these two minority populations in the context of different territorial opportunities and constraints. We discuss the major issues identified in the course of the research and themes such as our interlocutors' relationship with their faith at a time of *individual* need and *institutional* constraint, the 'religious welfarism' some of them proposed and the type of 'civic compliance' some also advanced.

6.2 Surviving the Storm: Religious Communities as Pandemic Welfare Providers in Milan

To cope with the exponential and dramatic increase in needs, strengthening state responsibility has been a key argument for launching of a large package of emergency investments in Italy (Pavolini et al., 2021) as in other European countries (Ferrera et al., 2022), such as lockdown benefits or wage subsidies. As often happens in a moment of crisis, the state's responsibility was emphasised but in this case there had been three decades of cuts and privatisations in the area of social policies, as well as populist, anti-state rhetoric in the name of freedom from the burden of money wasted on public services (Jessoula et al., 2022). National welfare systems, weakened by years of outsourcing and with inadequate safety nets, were not sufficiently ready to cover all the socio-economic risks that the pandemic created and/or intensified. However, significant help was provided by civil society organisations (CSOs), which supported state interventions through forms of partnership with local bureaucracies and public offices as well as through autonomous or networking aid initiatives.

The welfare role of religious associations, established by migrant minorities, has generally been neglected in both the literature and public debate concerning CSOs (Ambrosini et al., 2021a, 2021b). Their activism in terms of solidarity has become a pivotal core of their 'pandemic mission' (Molli, 2022), especially given the legal barriers[1] to accessing public welfare where migrants' social rights are often linked to their legal status and job position and given the lower economic incomes migrants often have at their disposal (Molli, 2018). Faced with these obstacles, religious leaders and activists

[1] See also 'When Institutions discriminate: Equality, Social Rights, Immigration'. Report of Project L.A.W.—Leverage the Access to Welfare: https://www.asgi.it/wp-content/uploads/2023/04/Report_LAW_EN.pdf.

among migrant minorities have developed complementary, alternative and often substitute services at both national and local level.

Our interlocutors provide a vivid insight into these issues. Carmen,[2] a woman who guides a Latin American group belonging to the main Milanese chaplaincy, worked to strengthen internal networks and provide various forms of help during the pandemic crisis:

> *This is our logic, and in the pandemic period we have tried to do this with chats and online communications, we write to each other and share information through the chats about needs and requirements ... The question of solidarity was important, we know that many people have lost their jobs, many ... Not only because they are 'badanti' or babysitters, but also others have lost their jobs ... So, I know what it means. We have motivated solidarity groups. Motivating groups is important, even a small gesture ... During the pandemic we gave a hand to others, we could not go out, and many of us were stuck at home, without assistance and without receiving a hand, many friends died. A woman I know was infected and stuck at home, we have friends around, Peruvians, we asked them ... and we have given them her number and they brought her some food for this lonely woman, first she didn't answer anyone on the phone, she was sick, then we succeeded, and we gave consolation. This is a case ... but I can say many, but many ... the situation got out of hand.*

Carmen operated as point of reference and confidant, since she understood the needs of her religious group and tried to find solutions. The example that Carmen provides in the interview clearly illustrates how 'pandemic counselling' played a significant role for those who did not have an extended family. Similarly, Marvin, a Catholic young man from El Salvador, who guides a religious unit linked to the same Milanese Catholic chaplaincy, has organised a series of helps mostly for irregular migrants, and he gives a vivid testimony of their living conditions:

> *Irregular immigrants are those who suffered the most, not just because of lack of work, also for a significant loss of money, if you are Italian you have priority ... but if you're without document what can you do? What can you do? A lot of us were without work, because the majority work as caregivers with elderly people, and some of them died by the way ... and so all these caregivers were without a job ... and without a permit in the midst of a pandemic ... Illegal immigrants suffered badly ... both economically and psychologically.*

[2] In the interests of anonymity we have given our interlocutors fictional names.

Faced with the critical situation of the pandemic community activists responded, and the priest of the chaplaincy provides an overview of the assistance being provided and their rationales:

> *I'd say a lot of internal solidarity. [I] consider that generally migrants are here with very few extended family relations ... some, maybe those who've been here the longest, but not the others. There's people here who needed support when they ended up in quarantine, many of them had no connections, and for others there are small families with no contacts with the outside ... There were people who took care of bringing them food and medicines, because nobody else could. It was a kind of spontaneous solidarity. They asked me to come and collect some basic things from the church [it being a centre for collecting goods] and they manage the rounds by themselves where they'd go out and help the families. Solidarity was important, at the basis of the help given. They collected boxes of food, they were well organised. I mean they didn't collect random stuff, but collected rationally what people needed, from food to medicines, because they knew the people, or they got the requests through other relations. They got organised to help one another.*

The immigrant Catholic chaplaincies supported people in a 'spirit of mutualism' that is grounded in a common identity and horizontal reciprocity. The ties between migrants, forged through religious attendance, created something like an 'extended family' that 'takes care of itself': what anthropologists also term as a 'fictive kinship' (Molli, 2020). In this sense, the call to 'your brother or sister as yourself' was the ethical compass that motivated their pandemic solidarity.

Despite these efforts, however, their welfare support has not been a panacea. Mutualism has encountered structural/physiological limits. It can provide basic support—so crucial during a moment of profound crisis—but could not cover all the pandemic risks. In this sense, the migrant Catholic chaplaincies worked in two main ways. They either provided the resources that members needed (mutualism) or communicated members' requests to the local Milanese charities (mediation). The chaplaincies functioned as hubs which filtered problems and acted as an extension of Italian Catholic associations such as Caritas, which could call on greater resources.

In the case of the Pentecostal Evangelical churches, the role of welfare was performed differently. Brenda, a young woman, tells how solidarity has de facto become a mission for the Latin American Pentecostal group to which she belongs:

> *We called all the members of the church and others contacted us, I can tell you we were contacted by a lot of families... and we gathered funds, and we received funds from a lot of places. Many were prepared to donate, and then we filtered through identifying critical cases inside the community. Consider I have a file of all the contacts, since I managed the helps for the brothers and sisters. I'd say at least 70 families from outside asked us for help. I mean 70 besides our church community [...] and we bought groceries.*

Her church reinterpreted its role as the pandemic 'calling it' to take action, both for the members and for other families in need. This Pentecostal community performed the welfare role as a form of 'mission in the city', addressing critical cases 'off the welfare's radar':

> *You have no idea ... During the first lockdown there was a family ... just to mention one case, they asked us help through Facebook. She said she needed help so we called her up to understand what she needed and she was crying and said she had nothing to feed her children with that night, an illegal immigrant, unemployed and with small children ... It was really hard for her. It was towards the end of the lockdown and the little savings she had were down to nothing and she had nothing left ... But people hold on—these are people that can resist, who are incredibly strong.*

So, religious congregations represented an 'alternative welfare hub' to which some families turned, especially in the case of the most vulnerable members of the migrant population. As Brenda explained during the interview, 'for these people the church became a central organization during the crisis, the entity which is closest in their lives'. Even if religious congregations could not provide the panacea for pandemic needs, their welfare commitment represented a precious support for the migrants' resilience.

6.3 The Role of Religious Communities as Civic Intermediators in Milan

Attitudes such as obedience and collaboration or criticism and scepticism in front of state decisions represent another key empirical focus for exploring the role of religious communities/identities during the pandemic crisis.

The restrictions imposed by state authorities raised a controversial normative question about the relationship between the state and religion and the reasons for public health security. This question referred to whether people should obey the *raison d'état* or assert religious freedom: both options were mutually exclusive during the pandemic. As we now know, the sanitary argument *de facto* prevailed in this normative hierarchy.

More precisely, the right to religious freedom as an absolute right remained but the ways in which it was concretely permitted and exercised were subject to various restrictions. In European countries, this coercion followed, despite some relevant differences in terms of restrictiveness (Mazurkiewicz, 2021), a common trend; there was a complete ban on collective worship during the first wave that often included the complete closure of religious sites and then a series of national accords allowing limited gatherings during the second and third wave.

Apart from the reactions by the historic religious denominations, which enjoyed institutional acknowledgement and well-defined channels of dialogue with national and local authorities, the reaction of migrant minorities represents an interesting issue, because they often lacked formal agreements and their settlement was often the target of prejudice and suspicion by many members of the receiving society. Requiring these minorities to comply with the pandemic regulations that were designed to both keep the 'situation under control' and promote civic contribution was not a matter of course. Moreover, 'loyalty to the state' was also affected by the fact that migrants were generally not the primary target of public welfare interventions. Indeed, at the beginning of the pandemic in Italy, foreigners were often blamed as 'spreaders of the virus' by populist forces.

The data, which we collected in Milan, enables us to explore the processes through which migrants from Peru and other Latin American countries responded to pandemic rules and addressed civic tasks. Although some criticisms emerged (in terms of a latent resistance), we saw evidence of both an active commitment and a diffused trust that could not be taken for granted. In Catholic churches, both religious and lay leaders encouraged worshippers to respect the guidelines and also provided specific information concerning members' situation to the authorities.

Our interview with a priest at a church, which had a large Latin American congregation, referred to the complete absence of the state beyond the official declaration of restrictions and described the reaction by members of the congregation:

> *The state ... the state didn't even see them [the migrants] ... I can say I expected this to happen, nothing new [...] because they are a weak class. What the state was especially unable to see—and this is very serious—was the medical implica-*

tions for all of those who didn't have an Italian health insurance card [irregular residents], because although it's true that if an immigrant goes to A&E [accident and emergency] he or she has a right to ad hoc assistance [that's to say that even as an illegal resident, the person is entitled to emergency assistance and is identified via the granting of a designated health insurance card/number] but if this isn't made clear people won't know, and this is serious lack of foresight …

The priest, drawing on his clerical status and taking advantage of well-established relations with authorities, initiated a series of institutional contacts by filtering the needs and preoccupations he perceived, such as in the specific case of irregular migrants:

I'll also tell you this—they (migrants) expected nothing from the state. They didn't even begin to think of it, and to tell you the truth, neither did I … apart from medicines … I mean when they [the illegal immigrants] started calling me saying they were scared to go out to the pharmacy, and that's when I started worrying. So, through institutional and personal contacts I said to the people in the high places [members of the Ministry of Interior] I said, you need to send a strong message to say that … Their answer was that this couldn't be done but tell them [the immigrants] that they can rest assured … not to worry … And so I told everyone not to worry … 'We are in Italy.' And anyway how would they manage a deportation when everything was stuck? But you know how it is when you're scared … It difficult to change someone's mind if they're scared.

He was conscious that panic and fear inevitably emerge during a liminal period, especially when public institutions do not help migrant minorities and their life-conditions. As he commented during the interview 'communicating calmly to them was difficult. They were scared'. In this sense, the Catholic community compensated for the state's absence and served as a point of reference for diffusing information on how to deal with pandemic restrictions.

The process, however, was not always easy, especially after the first prolonged lockdown. Strong ethnic and social cohesion underpins the establishment of religious congregations abroad but this can make the role of a religious leader difficult. The priest narrates how he also became a sort of policeman confronted with the feelings that developed among worshippers who wanted to freely meet their brothers and sisters:

[Interviewer] How do they perceive danger?

[Priest] Yes, foolishness and the inability to handle feelings. They think we are … we are cold as worshippers [we don't express as they do religious fervour and a certain kind of participation during Mass]. On Sundays a typical scene is when I demand for the safe distancing to be respected … I say: 'Don't get too close together' … and then outside when they are leaving they're all hugging and kissing, And so I say: 'Brothers and sisters, what you do outside is not my responsibility but don't stand so close together in front of the saints.' But when you speak to Peruvians … you know what they are like, Samuele … you've seen them, they all have to pray and they all want to light a candle for El signor del Milagros … And if you tell them anything else someone will think that the parish priest is a man of little faith … who doesn't protect them while they are there praying.

Catholic chaplains, therefore, reinterpreted their role and mandate during the pandemic, alternating between representing migrants' demands to the authorities and keeping them in line with state regulations.

Pentecostal activists developed similar practices in terms of civic engagement. As we have seen, their solidarity activism became a mission in Milan, and they also disseminated pandemic news to fellow worshippers:

There was always someone from the church who'd translate the information (guidelines and restrictions) into Spanish, plus we used Whatsapp groups and created posters to go round on the Internet and in chat rooms, everybody was informed and we also managed to reach those who had no social networks available, and we called on them at home to tell them what they should and shouldn't do. We contacted all of them and other people too. We always warned the brothers and sisters of the community, you know … Explaining things is not always that easy … Think of older people … they ask you: 'Why can't we go to the market?' And it wasn't easy to explain the type of risk they'd be running.

As Brenda, a young woman, explained during the interview, the church started to act in a 'capillary way'. They contacted all the members and translated the regulations, making them easier to understand. Also Rafael, a volunteer leader at another Evangelical church involved in the study, tells how his church performed the same role:

I would say that the state … how should I put it?—we mainly took it onto ourselves to help each other out. With respect to information, let's say that we shared information via Zoom, especially for permits necessary in order to leave your house—many didn't know how it was done. And so thanks to community ties we

> *shared information. Then there was a period when they gave a permit for going to church service [while in the first phase of the pandemic the churches were closed], and then we shared the information about how to get a permit to go to church to pray ... for us it was important. There was a lot of information going around, and through acquaintances we clarified the information. If I had any doubts I would ask an Italian Baptist Church, because they have a lawyer. And so we knew how to go about things properly without making mistakes—we asked them how to behave if in doubt.*

The attitudes of both Brenda's and Rafael's churches may appear exemplary. They performed—probably better than the Catholic communities—a role of 'civicness' in relation to the decisions of the public authorities. In this sense, Pentecostals worked to spread a sense of self-discipline and self-control in front of chaos and anomie, although none of these religious communities are officially recognised by the state and lack any official recognition by local institutions. This can also be interpreted as a 'strategy'—namely, a willingness to demonstrate responsibility as well as to demonstrate that they 'deserve' acknowledgement. In this sense, presenting themselves as 'allies of the state' can be also conceived as a tool to try to create preconditions for a new recognition.

The communities we studied not only functioned as civic intermediaries but also directly sponsored civic activities. Some worshippers decided to promote forms of support not only for their members but also for the local community where the respective church is located or in neighbourhoods where they themselves lived, showing a sense of empathy with the Italian society:

> *Those who are more inside and have been here the longest, with contacts in the territory, some of them did voluntary work, you know ... In the various neighbourhoods there was a need to help the elderly, those in quarantine, those who were frightened and refused to go out. They were simple but important forms of help.*

As the Catholic priest explains, some decided to volunteer during the pandemic through micro-acts of solidarity that were important because they came from a population not particularly wealthy in socio-economic terms and which, often, is socially stigmatised. Similarly, Brenda explains how her group organised not only for themselves but for the local territory some forms of help:

> *Some of our group also helped as best they could. They got organized. And if someone from the neighbourhood was sick or stuck at home they'd go out and do the shopping for them. There was both effort and predisposition. Those who had the opportunity would do what they could in their neighbourhood. You know … little things but useful ones: the shopping, visiting older people, asking if anyone needed help…*

'Little things but useful' synthesises this solidarity predisposition, and it was not limited to the case studies considered during our project. Many Catholic chaplaincies in Lombardy and Pentecostal churches have organised collections for Italian charities, in Milan, Como and Bergamo, for example, and for the respective city hospital, showing 'empathy and engagement' for what was a critical situation.

6.4 The Role of Mosques During the Pandemic: The Case of the Brick Lane Mosque

Mosques also played a crucial role in mediating between the state and migrant minorities in Britain and London, in particular. Despite the many similarities in the way governments in both countries reacted to the pandemic, religious diversity was more formally accepted in the British public arena. The Board of Deputies of British Jews was founded in 1760 to represent Jewish citizens at the national level while the Muslim Council of Britain, founded in 1997, was the 'UK's largest Muslim umbrella organisation with over 500 members including mosques, schools, charitable associations and professional networks'.[3] At the local level a wide range of non-Christian religious centres had developed to serve the needs of Jews, Muslims, Hindus, Sikhs, Jains and Buddhists, while a number of private educational institutions had also emerged such as madrassahs and Islamic secondary schools.

One of the ten 'experts', whom Shamea Mia interviewed, was an imam at the Brick Lane Mosque. The mosque represented vividly the history of immigration and cultural diversity that characterised this area of London. It was housed within a building which began life as a Christian chapel erected by French Protestant refugees who had settled in the area during the late seventeenth and early eighteenth centuries. When Polish and Russian Jews settled here during the late nineteenth century, it served as a

[3] https://mcb.org.uk/purpose/ accessed 4/7/2023.

synagogue and Talmudic school, and after the arrival of Bangladeshi migrants during the 1960s and 1970s it was turned into a mosque.

The interview was undertaken at the mosque during December 2021. It was conducted in Bengali and then transcribed by Shamea Mia. By the time the interview took place there had been two lockdowns and restrictions on social interaction but as the vaccination programme got underway during the autumn of 2021 the health emergency was starting to weaken. In the interview, therefore, the imam was invited to reflect on what had been happening locally, how the operation of the mosque had been affected and the impact on people's religious beliefs and practices.

The mosque had conformed with government regulations and closed during the lockdowns. Reflecting on the easing of restrictions after the first lockdown, the imam explained that:

> *We had to manage people in a way so that they did not mix ... but thanks to the Almighty that we were able to manage it during this time ... We did not maintain a timetable during the pandemic either—so we kept the mosque open for 24 hours.*

The imam and others involved in managing the mosque acted as important monitors of what was happening across the neighbourhood by checking on what may have happened to regular worshippers:

> *When people pray their five daily prayers, we see them five times a day. But when we didn't see people coming to the mosque, who came regularly, we wondered what happened to them ... This feeling of congregation in prayer is a great benefit for the community ... And it was a good way of finding out information, that people will ask about you and this is how we found out about each other ... And, of course, it is the digital age, so people call each other up and tell each other about their problems ... And we also announced that if people are in difficulty, please get in touch with us ... So we tried to the best of our ability*

The imam also reflected on how people had reacted to the pandemic in religious terms and the fears it had instilled in them:

> *As a Muslim community, we believe sometimes the Almighty tests us and we found that people were a bit more fearful now. Of course, we can't say how long this fear of God will last but some sort of fear has been instilled that perhaps the pandemic has happened because we have sinned and this is the wrath of the Almighty. Or what will happen once we die? And this has had an effect on the community.*

Like the purpose-built East London Mosque nearby, the Brick Lane Mosque was very much in the public eye and so the imam and others involved in the management of the building had to be very careful about observing state regulations. Both mosques served as more than just religious centres. As the imam himself noted: 'the mosque is a communal meeting place as well as a place for worship'. Other community activists were also well aware of the political effect of mosques not conforming as we have seen in the chapter on Tower Hamlets where the borough councillor, Irfan Iqbal, commented about the danger of not 'playing the game' and how the 'Muslim community' could be blamed for any large outbreak of the virus.

6.5 The Impact of the 2020 Lockdown on Religious Life

The March 2020 lockdown had an immediate impact on Christian, Hindu, Sikh, Buddhist and Muslim religious observance and their ritual calendars. In the case of Bangladeshi Muslims in Tower Hamlets, the performance of the daily prayers at local mosques was suspended and this largely affected male worshippers since they attended mosques in much larger numbers than women. The caretaker of the Brick Lane Mosque, Asad Chowdhury, was keenly aware of the social function that the mosque served:

> *When you see people, it gives you a strength to live longer because that means they can exchange views, how family are doing, sharing opinions etc … But when people are solely alone … they beg to meet with people … When people go to a religious place, they feel empowered.*

He had the difficult task of ensuring that the official regulations were observed. He had to stand at the entrance door, take people's temperatures and then stop anyone with a high temperature attending prayers:

> *There were a few people who would say: 'Let me in' … but I would show them their temperature and [say]: 'You're not allowed in … If this happened to me, I would also not be allowed in … Please don't mind but please contact the doctor, who will be able to help you and it will be good for you' … Some people got angry but I smiled and laughed and told them as best as I could … And there were some people who wouldn't listen and community members came to help.*

As Irfan Iqbal explained, praying in the various mosques that had sprung up in Tower Hamlets was very important for many elderly male residents:

A lot of elderly people I know want to live and remain in Tower Hamlets because they can easily access religious activities ... meaning mosque activities... including my own father ... I lost my father in 2010, but we couldn't convince him to move out of where he was living ... He was living just 100 yards from East London Mosque so you can imagine... There are people of that sort, they can afford and are able but they won't move out of the area because they are so used to and they wanted to be part of that essential [facility] ... To some, they might not regard religious activities as essential but to our elderly generation, they regard religious activities as part of their integral living or essential that they need to access and go to everyday.

The month of fasting during Ramadan and the celebration of Eid ul-Fitr at the end of Ramadan also could not be observed in the usual way. Drawing on his youth work, Irfan Iqbal was particularly interested in the impact on young people:

So we went through the sort of whole Ramadan thing ... and people couldn't pray the late night prayers ... That affects [people] a lot of the time as well ... Because when you're 15, 16, 17, you go to late night prayers, you do bits of it, then you go out with your friends, late night, come back to the mosque ... And it's part of growing up but you miss all of that.

Eid al-Fitr is celebrated both publicly and at home and normally lasts several days:

[It] features two to three days of celebrations that include special morning prayers. People greet each other with "Eid Mubarak," meaning "Blessed Eid" and with formal embraces. Sweet dishes are prepared at home and gifts are given to children and to those in need. In addition, Muslims are encouraged to forgive and seek forgiveness.[4]

Government restrictions on social interaction, such as the 'rule of six', that followed the strict lockdown presented the local borough council with a difficult political dilemma as Irfan Iqbal noted:

[4] https://dornsife.usc.edu/news/stories/what-is-eid-al-fitr/#:~:text=Eid%20al%2DFitr%20means%20%E2%80%9Cthe,to%20sundown%20for%20a%20month.

I think the first time they had sort of prayers outside, people are gathering outside they just wanted to do the Eid prayers… and people were, sort of like, in a sort of gathering and saying, like: 'No [restrictions].' … I remember I spoke to the mayor about it … 'So what can you do about it?' … He was like, you know: 'What do we do?' [I said]: 'You know, if people want to pray outside, say, you know, in a car park 50, 100 people get together … okay, do we go there full force and stop the religious act?'

The mayor decided that discretion was the better part of valour and chose to turn a blind eye.

6.6 Mortality During the Pandemic: The Role of the Brisk Lane Mosque

Asad Chowdhury and the imam were intimately involved in maintaining the traditional funeral rituals at the mosque. Asad Chowdhury explained what happened during the worst stage of the pandemic when many people were dying:

There is still a need to look after the building and maintain it, and there are so many dead bodies coming in and people dying … lots of Bangladeshis …They came and we read the Janazah prayers … People came and, say, used the toilet or performed ablutions to prepare for the Janazah … So there was a need for extra people to come and work and I sorted this all out … There were so many… We had 8, 10, 12 bodies in one go and we had 6 to 8 bodies daily … People washed the bodies and those who had families, the families came … those who died from the virus. They were afraid … and they couldn't see the body.

He explained that the washing of the bodies was a gendered process:

There was a specific person who came, who is the manager and supervised everyone. So the men washed the men's bodies and the women washed the women's bodies … After the washing, they'd be put into the morgue and the Janazah would be prayed and there would be a lot of prayers prayed and, lastly, the bodies would be taken to where they would be laid to rest.

The imam also movingly spoke about the inability to grieve during the height of the pandemic in 2020:

The situation was such that people couldn't express their grief during the pandemic, there wasn't any scope for that, someone came with the body of their father, washed the body and prayed the Janazah in half an hour and the then the body was taken to be buried ... he doesn't have time to express his grief ... It was a very sad time ... Lots of people didn't know find out about their close friends' deaths during lockdown, they found out after ... they didn't know friends had passed away, it was just close family who knew ... not even the whole extended family knew sometimes ... Initially, the body was sealed in the hospital and then taken directly to the cemetery ... This was definitely a very sad time that we passed through.

6.7 Conclusion

This chapter has explored the ways in which religion played a crucial intermediary role for minority populations during the global health crisis as well as its socio-economic consequences. We began by focusing on political and legal factors as these shaped the official recognition of migrants from different religious backgrounds, how migrants operated in the public sphere and how they criticised or made requests to local authorities. Hence, the ways in which religions have incorporated and reinterpreted the onset of the pandemic and the restrictions on social interaction were also influenced by the degree of political and social recognition they had acquired during their settlement in a new country.

We also explored the symbolic dimensions of the emergency guidelines since these guidelines raise an epistemological/ontological question about which types of values should be prioritised during a crisis. As we know, biomedical and economic arguments prevailed and, therefore, one of the major issues raised in this chapter was the conflict between those arguments and the religious principles avowed by these minorities. We then proceeded to explore how the minorities developed a local-level perspective towards their concrete experiences at the time of the pandemic. Some of the issues we identified are transversal, while others apply specifically to either Milan or London.

In Milan, 'religious welfarism' was a key process, which reflected the crucial social role that Roman Catholic chaplaincies played in the life of Latin American residents beyond such pull factors as culture and language. During the crisis, these chaplaincies relaunched and redesigned their roles in order to support and foster solidarity. Internal networks were rapidly activated through the collection of funds and they have operated as a filter that linked members' needs to other Catholic charities. For the Pentecostals, welfare provision has instead become a 'mission' where providing for the needy represented a key task and a sort of theological call—in terms of an eschatology of the pandemic—for identifying souls in need in Milan. Catholic and Pentecostal churches, therefore, were pivotal—especially during the first lockdown—in addressing the key weaknesses in Italian social and welfare provision. The issue of religious welfarism also appears in the London study and highlights the profound relation between religion and solidarity. In this sense, religious hubs during the pandemic compensated for the state's limitations at the local level.

Another issue concerned people's compliance with restrictions, and here there were some differences between the Milan and London. In Milan, the Roman Catholic priest and lay leaders were conscious of the panic that could emerge during a period of great insecurity and sought to encourage calm and foster trust through their role as mediators between the congregants and the authorities. This strategy drew on the good general relationship between the Catholic Church and public institutions in Italy. However, the work of the ethnic chaplaincies shows that this relationship should not be taken for granted since disorientation and problems were many and various and the process of encouraging compliance was not always direct and easy.

Pentecostal activists operated in a similar way with regard to civic engagement. Because their activities still lack any formal recognition by local state institutions, we interpreted Pentecostal activism as a strategy for demonstrating responsibility, the capacity of self-control and, thus, their deservedness for a (possible) future recognition. As a young female leader declared: 'we want to stay regular even if we are irregular'. However, because some members were 'illegals'—they did not have official documents—avoiding any involvement with the state was crucial for them. We cannot generalise from our case study for Pentecostal churches across Italy and elsewhere but it was clear that in Milan at least the pandemic created a choice—stay close to the state or stay with God.

In terms of civic engagement, both Catholic and Pentecostal minorities have promoted forms of volunteering within local neighbourhoods through micro-acts of solidarity. It is important to acknowledge these micro-acts since they came from a population that was hit hard by the pandemic and was often stigmatised as 'scroungers' of welfare services in populist rhetoric.

The issue of civic engagement was also a key theme in London. Although official restrictions had a major impact on the social and cultural life of local Bangladeshis, those based at local mosques sought to encourage trust in state pronouncements and regulations. Bangladeshi responses were not uniform, however, and were shaped by the ways in which people balanced the value of their customs/traditions against state restrictions.

As for the post-pandemic future, our research raises the question whether state institutions have learned anything from their engagement with those, who represented minority religious congregations during the pandemic. Some dialogue did indeed develop at the local level but it now seems that this dialogue has taken the form of 'failed promises'. Minorities have demonstrated, along with their ability to react, considerable flexibility when confronted with political and social contingences but it is an open question whether state institutions can show the same flexibility and engage more closely and effectively with minorities.

References

Ambrosini, M., Bonizzoni, P., & Molli, S. D. (2021a). How Religion Shapes Immigrants' Integration: The Case of Christian Migrant Churches in Italy. *Current Sociology, 69*(6), 823–842.

Ambrosini, M., Bonizzoni, P., & Molli, S. D. (2021b). Il welfare informale dei migranti. Chiese etniche e processi di inclusione sociale a Milano. *Rassegna Italiana di Sociologia, 62*(1), 165–196.

Ambrosini, M., Molli, S. D., & Naso, P. (2022). *Quando gli immigrati vogliono pregare. Comunità, pluralismo, welfare.* Il Mulino.

Barbalet, J., Possamai, A., & Turner, B. S. (2011). *Religion and the State: A Comparative Sociology.* Anthem Press.

Bonizzoni, P., & Dotsey, S. (2021). Migration and Legal Precarity in the Time of Pandemic: Qualitative Research on the Italian Case. *Dve Domovini, 54*, 117–130.

Colombo, E. (2021). Human Rights-inspired Governmentality: COVID-19 through a Human Dignity Perspective. *Critical Sociology, 47*(4–5), 571–581.

Connor, P. (2012). Balm for the Soul: Immigrant Religion and Emotional Well-being. *International Migration, 50*(2), 130–157.

Del Re, E., & Naso, P. (2022). *Religioni e pandemia in Italia. Dottrina, comunità, cura.* Rubettino.

Eade, J. (2011). From Race to Religion: Multiculturalism and Contested Urban Space. In J. Beaumont & C. Baker (Eds.), *Postsecular Cities: Space, Theory and Practice* (pp. 154–167). Continuum.

Ferrera, M., Miró, J., & Ronchi, S. (2022). Walking the Road Together? EU Polity Maintenance During the COVID-19 Crisis. *West European Politics, 44*(5–6), 1329–1352.

Giordan, G., & Palmisano, S. (2022). Introduzione: La religione ai tempi del Coronavirus. *Religioni e Società, XXXVII, 103*, 10–13.

Hirschman, C. (2004). The Role of Religion in the Origins and Adaptation of Immigrant Groups in the United States. *International Migration Review, 38*(3), 1206–1233.

Jessoula, M., Natili, M., & Pavolini, N. (2022). 'Exclusionary Welfarism': A New Programmatic Agenda for Populist Right-wing Parties? *Contemporary Politics, 28*(4), 447–468.

Levitt, P. (2007). *God Needs No Passport*. The New Press.

Maestripieri, L. (2021). The Covid-19 Pandemics: Why Intersectionality Matters. *Frontiers in sociology, 6*, 642–662.

Mazurkiewicz, P. (2021). Religious Freedom in the Time of the Pandemic. *Religions, 12*(2), 103.

Molli, S. D. (2018). *Gli stranieri stanno bene. Salute e integrazione degli immigrati*. ITL.

Molli, S. D. (2020). Immigrant Religious Networks in Milan: Ethnic Churches as Source of Social Capital. *Mondi Migranti, 1*, 97–116.

Molli, S. D. (2022). Immigrant Women's Protagonism: Exercising Leadership Roles in Ethnic Churches at the Time of the Pandemic in Italy. *Religions, 13*(8), 696.

Molteni, F., Landini, R., Biolcati, F., Chiesi, A. M., Dotti Sani, G. M., Guglielmi, S., Maraffi, M., Pedrazzani, A., Segatti, P., & Vezzoni, C. (2021). Searching for Comfort in Religion: Insecurity and Religious Behaviour During the COVID-19 Pandemic in Italy. *European Societies, 23*(1), 704–720.

Pace, E. (2021). Il respiro corto dello Spirito nelle mega-chiese, ai tempi della pandemia. *Comparative Cultural Studies-European and Latin American Perspectives, 6*(13), 21–35.

Pastore, F. (2021). Migrazioni e pandemia: interazioni empiriche e spunti teorici. *Mondi Migranti, 1*, 19–43.

Pavolini, E., Sabatinelli, S., & Vesan, P. (2021). I servizi di welfare in Italia alla prova della pandemia. Uno sguardo di insieme. *Social Policies, 8*(2), 211–232.

Ricucci, R., & Bossi, L. (2022). From Collectivities to Families and Back to the Individual: Religiosity, Migrations and Civic Engagement at the Beginning of the COVID Period in a Multicultural Italian City. *Religions, 13*(6), 497.

CHAPTER 7

The Importance of Urban Culture as a Middle Ground Between State and Ethnic Minorities in Negotiating (Im)mobilities: The London Context

Shamea Y. Mia

7.1 Introduction

What might it mean to negotiate a sense of personal space within an urban context? The complexities of factors such as class and gender are involved when trying to situate oneself within the urban dynamic. However, cultural dynamics and ongoing cultural change also play a crucial role as well as feelings about belonging to differing cultural traditions that can potentially impact the position one occupies in the city. This chapter will explore these issues in the context of the Bangladeshi diasporic population in Tower Hamlets during the COVID-19 pandemic and connected issues involving technological spaces, communication and freedoms, the impact

S. Y. Mia (✉)
University of Roehampton, London, UK
e-mail: symia@hotmail.com

M. Caselli et al. (eds.), *Migrants' (Im)mobilities in Three European Urban Contexts*, Europe in a Global Context,
https://doi.org/10.1007/978-3-031-53773-8_7

of belonging to local social networks and the overarching structural systems that affect our interactions with institutions. Although our project engaged with members of different migrant groups in three European cities, we will focus mainly on the London case.

7.2 The 'Entirety' of Tower Hamlets

In understanding the lives and experiences of our interlocutors in the London borough of Tower Hamlets, it is important to understand three interconnected levels; the macro level (official government bodies and the healthcare system, for instance), the meso level (the crucial in-between component between the macro and micro levels) and the micro level (the everyday lives of 'ordinary' citizens in the borough and their experiences). In terms of theory, the model of social systems will be utilised to analyse the relationship between the three levels (Serpa & Ferreira, 2019; Sampson, 1991; Bergström & Dekker, 2014). Substantively, this chapter will focus on how identities and belongings are negotiated and re-negotiated in relation to these systems, as expressed through the voices of our interlocutors.

Bentley's (2020) diagram in Fig. 7.1 shows the interlinking of multi-factorial facets that exacerbate the risks of infection and death for ethnic

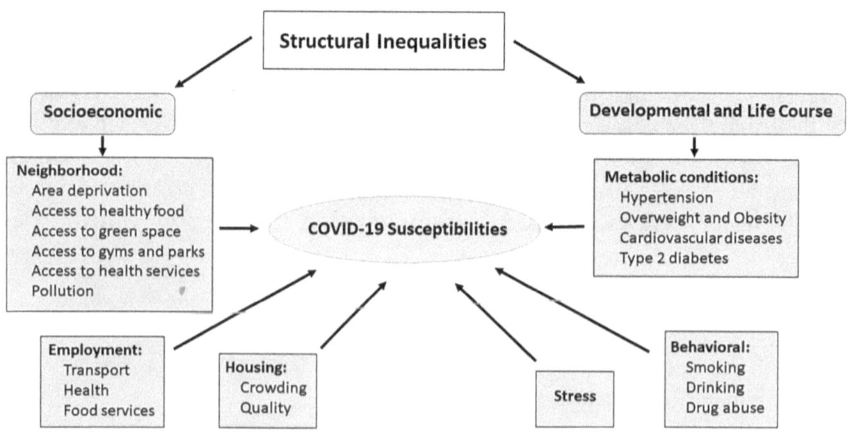

Fig. 7.1 The relationship of structural inequalities to susceptibility to COVID-19 (Bentley, 2020)

minority groups from COVID-19, i.e. the socio-economic factors and the underlying health factors that potentially contributed to COVID-19 infections.

When discussing how those in London are embedded in the multi-layered and complex tapestries of their geographical locale, it is important to bear in mind that ideas around belonging and identity are closely linked to ethnicity. As Baumann (1999) notes, ethnicity is not a 'natural' identity but is cultivated and often used as a means or a strategy for social action. Gilroy (2006) also suggests that power and authority are involved when a group wants to understand itself in terms of identity. Indeed, this is especially important as ethnicity can become a means of political engagement.

Citizens and spaces are not fixed but are in constant flux. The experience of migrants is particularly telling here since they are linked to both their countries of origin and their countries of destination. Anthias (2009), for example, has highlighted the complexities of what she describes as 'transnational actors' and the need to move away from fixed spatial boundaries to understand the intersectionalities of ethnicity, gender, generation and class. As we shall see later in this chapter, our interlocutors identify as Bangladeshi but sometimes in very different ways. They come from different generations and have been affected by the pandemic in different ways. They identify as male or female and demonstrate different levels of religiosity and ethnic belonging.

Hence, when thinking about *where* our interlocutors fit into the greater system highlighted by Bentley's (2020) diagram above, we must bear in mind that the COVID pandemic often brought people in various local networks together through language, religion, personal experiences, ties with other people and culture. As Werbner (2005) notes, culture is embodied in rituals, performances and social exchanges and the pandemic has taught us that multicultural citizenship is responsive, inventive and ever changing (see also Werbner, 2010). This means that the Bangladeshi cultural influences evident in Tower Hamlets are by no means static and immovable, but are in constant flux, dynamic and enterprising as we shall hear in our encounters with our interlocutors.

In this chapter we will hear stories about the role that mosques played, not only as places of religious worship but also as social venues where different generations could come together to talk about life experiences in safe and familiar settings. Moreover, through the intervention of local Bangladeshi doctors, mosques were also spaces where health issues could be discussed and vaccine hesitancy dispelled. Imams and mosque committee members were in close contact with medical professionals and local government officials and worked to solve urgent issues around vaccine uptake and health and wellbeing.

With regard to the systems perspective introduced above, the diagram in Fig. 7.2 portrays the position of the meso level and the crucial role it played in relaying information between official institutions and local residents and interpreting people's positionalities, where it proved to be an important site for community engagement, since it included local councillors, social influencers, leaders of community organisations, imams and providers of services such as funeral directors. It therefore acted as a platform for various actors' agency and resilience, some of whose voices will be heard later in this chapter.

During 2021, the Tower Hamlets borough council had introduced Covid Champions who acted as an important link between government institutions and the NHS and local residents. We hear one of their voices below.

> *[Interviewer] So, tell me about some of the work that you do as a Covid Champion*
>
> *[Respondent] ... when Covid came about, none of us knew what we were going to do... there was a bit of uncertainty at the beginning ... but (then) a lot of us got together and we had worked for Tower Hamlets for a long time and there were those who were over 50 and had the most problems, there was panic buying and people didn't want to leave their homes ... and we worked mainly with Bengalis, who didn't leave their homes because of fear (unclear) ... We*

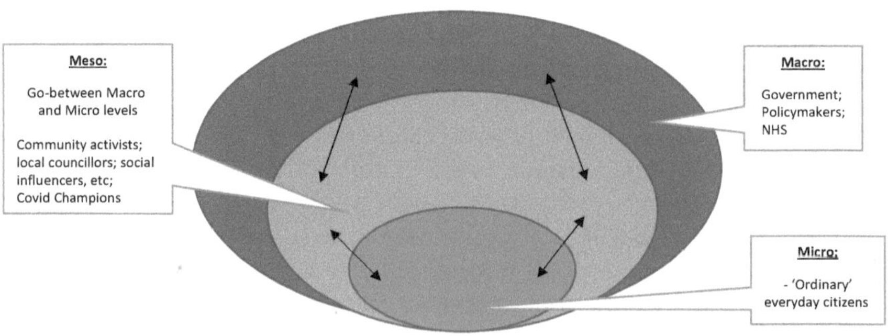

Fig. 7.2 An overview of interrelationships for the London borough of Tower Hamlets between the Macro, Meso and Micro levels

worked in teams and we went to people's houses … lots of people didn't have rice, groceries, shopping or medicines … there are lots of people who live alone, who don't have a son or a daughter, say … they have no-one and can't go out … we helped over 100 individuals and families, mainly in Tower Hamlets …In the beginning, we gave out free masks … then we helped with shopping, people would give us their money to do the shopping for them and we would deliver it to them … I have a car … We would deliver medicines as well … Some people can't cook, so we would order food for them … We did whatever we could to help people … Different people did different things … There were about 50, 60 of us Covid Champions working together … There are about 50,000 people living here … so we couldn't help everyone … When people wanted to see their children, we took them to see them from outside, 10, 15 minutes or half an hour, then back. This we did for free.

We see from the above extract how Covid Champions helped their own social networks as well as others during the crisis. Most of those, who were helped by our interlocutor, were Bangladeshis, reflecting the important presence of the Bangladeshi diaspora in this area of London.

We can see from the narrative above how many among the Bangladeshi diaspora in Tower Hamlets were helped to adapt to the novel ways of living during and after the COVID-19 pandemic. The respondent's contribution to society as a Covid Champion reflects the cohesion within Bangladeshi networks across this area of London, and it also demonstrates the importance of the meso level to understanding how people were helped to access the various services provided by the borough. As Frink et al. (2008) argue, there is accountability at the meso level, where organisations answer to others. At the governmental level, people's behaviour was regulated in terms of not going out through the various lockdowns or being encouraged to engage with the vaccination programme, for example. However, these official measures and promotions relied on mediation through the meso level, where there was more scope to influence individuals at the micro level and feed this back to the macro level. Those, who operated at this level, became responsible for imparting knowledge, therefore, and their role helps us to understand from a system's perspective the wider implications of operating at the meso level and the relationship this level has with the other two levels. Without the meso level, the relationship between the micro and the macro levels would have been less efficient.

7.3 Elastic Networked Systems

If we think about the aforementioned system as fluid and dynamic, we can argue that there is movement and fluidity between the levels as well. This can be seen in terms of actors within the network changing their roles and adapting to new situations as we will see below. The evidence of changing roles and fluidity is also important when bearing in mind the relationship between the interviewer and the respondent, especially when language and traditions are shared. Interlocutors were able to air their experiences, fears and observations with me as a researcher on the project, since I shared a similar cultural heritage and language (at times, the interviews were conducted in Bengali and translated during transcription). This often allowed me to be more quickly accepted into their own social networks and considerably helped the snowballing process.

At the micro level there was also an element of elasticity, which enabled social actors to change tack or manoeuvre to a certain degree within the system. If we think of those operating at different levels of the system as members of changing, flexible 'networks' rather than as contained within static, bounded 'communities', it is easier to see how people relate to and position themselves within such systems. Individuals feel that they are somehow connected to each other in various ways but through a social construction that is imagined (Anderson, 2006). Structures are still important and play an important role at the macro level of government and healthcare institutions, for example, but this level operates in the background and allows for a certain degree of flexibility within the structural system. When this flexibility is forcefully taken away—as with the stringent lockdown during the COVID-19 pandemic—and individuals are faced with no choice except to follow orders handed down from the macro level, there is an impact upon an individual's peace of mind, as we shall hear later in this chapter.

7.4 Technology, Bangladeshis and the COVID-19 Pandemic in London

Being stuck at home during the lockdowns and being obliged to conduct social or work activities online (the lack of access to virtual communications will be discussed later) had two major consequences. People were usually in comfortable surroundings that were familiar and could save the time and cost of travelling to work. They often also shared a space with another human being and this enabled them a degree of intimacy that was much more intense than online communication:

> *Initially, I was not familiar with Zoom and a lot of other people were not familiar with Zoom … but when I realised the potentiality of Zoom, it was very exciting that you don't have to leave your home … saving money and time … (But) the atmosphere and the interaction you get in a physical meeting is very different … physical meetings are needed as well (as online ones) otherwise you cannot do the general things … You don't have the personal touch.*

In many ways connectedness became a central feature of the pandemic and the need for human interaction became more urgent (Nitschke et al., 2021; De' et al., 2020). Technology enabled people to connect to others across the globe in a digital space which, despite great distances, brought people in greater proximity to each other. Phones, laptops and other devices became more important as a means for communication when people did not have the freedom to move in open spaces. Yet, as the above quote indicates, whilst time and money were saved, people missed the physical connectedness of each other—the tactile touch that influences how we interact with each other, eye contact, hand-shaking, physical closeness when we sit together—all of these little intimacies, which we have with each other, became lost in the digital space. As Sommerlad et al. (2022) have shown, those who had more quality face-to-face or phone and/or video contact with others were less prone to depression, while people who were sociable and forced into lockdown had higher depressive symptoms.

Digital communication did allow people, who were not physically present, to be present in a virtual landscape and see loved ones, who were both present and not present at the same time. This is described below when our interlocutor spoke about conducting the funeral rites of a parent who had passed away:

> *I did a lot of my funeral arrangements on video calling … and WhatsApp … At the same time you have to remember that we're working with people who aren't used to these [video] platforms … A lot of families were used to things like WhatsApp … [so] WhatsApp was brilliant in terms of using the video. [Through] that platform you could bring, say, three people on and that really worked well … We were doing face to face consultations and, say, if a family member was from across the world, we wouldn't normally invite them for a meeting because we wouldn't have this but then, because we'd had this practice of inviting different parts of the world to the meeting, that means they can be present especially in the second lockdown.*

> *So we diversified and got creative in many ways … I remember doing a funeral last January and, um, … we had the son here and we had the other son on camera on another phone and we had the sister from Dubai on another phone. So that meant all three siblings could partake in the arrangements of their father's funeral but normally, it would be just that one person.*

It appears that the pandemic led to a more streamlining and seamless interaction with others, especially in the digital realm (Wolhuter & Jacobs, 2021) on the revolutionising effects on using digital platforms in the education industry, for instance. As we can see from the quote above, digital communications were particularly useful for some businesses, making it much quicker and easier to get the job done. The same interlocutor describes how the bureaucratic process involved in registering deaths was streamlined:

> *A lot of our work has to do with legal paperwork, but all that's been digitalised now, so before people had to go and physically register a death … and that's all gone now … so there have been lots of parts of the legal side of it has been really fast tracked and been made much easier and us, we're having to basically keep up with it, so there have been lots and lots of changes and I would say there's been change for the better because it was quite archaic … What the pandemic did was make everyone become technologically aligned.*

Digitalisation enabled the institutional system to cope with the increased number of people dying during the pandemic, and for this interlocutor, this was a positive outcome of the pandemic. It could also be argued that the efficiency of the digital platform strengthened the relationship between the micro and macro levels because it allowed for easier access and communication between different parties at the meso level where the legal paperwork occurred.

Yet, as we have mentioned before, not everyone had access to technology and this exacerbated the social inequalities that became very evident during the COVID-19 pandemic (see Beaunoyer et al., 2020). As a local borough councillor commented:

> *We noticed that people weren't engaging much, so digitally, we tried to engage young people, especially the younger ages in school or so, but then you actually figure out that there's a whole dimension of digital exclusion happening as well … So families on the poverty line or not doing well financially if they have two or three kids and, um, they probably have one device … A lot of the time it's*

their Mum's or Dad's mobile phone or probably one device and they're having to share between two or three people so the exclusion was quite real.

The digital divide particularly affects the elder minority ethnic population (see Poole et al., 2021) and this was starkly evident from our own study. The elderly were forced to stay inside and many were unable to access or use the Internet unless there was someone who lived in the same household and was Internet literate. Indeed, for elderly Bangladeshi males being unable to pursue social activities such as going to the local mosque, where they might meet friends and enquire about others, had a detrimental effect on both their physical and mental health:

[Respondent] I think the coronavirus has directly and indirectly affected all of us ... Older people more than younger people because they had to spend more time indoors as opposed to doing any kind of activity including visiting the mosque ... The mosque has always been a place of socialisation for the vast majority of the Muslim elderly ... This is where they go to meet up with their friends, pray, have a little chitchat and come home ... but that was taken away ... for compulsory reasons... I think because of the pandemic, because of their vulnerability, they were not able to access the essential healthcare services ... Remotely accessing and face to face accessing are totally different.

[Interviewer] Ok, so by remotely accessing, what do you mean by that? By means of the internet?

[Respondent] By the internet, or the telephone or mobile phone and quite a lot of the time especially with elderly people ... and with our people, unless you are in a position to establish rapport, you would hardly be in a position to get anything out of them ... So spending a couple of minutes on the phone, how much rapport can a clinician or a health professional would be able to establish?... If you are treating with someone who is elderly, you need to spend a lot of time establishing some sort of social rapport in order for them to open up and discuss their problems openly and honestly ... especially with our people, because of the culture with which we have immigrated or our cultural background, it's quite difficult.

Rapport, therefore, was seen as crucial in engaging with the elder generation for the above interlocutor and research indicates that the frailer citizens were during the pandemic, the higher number of consultations they needed (Joy et al., 2020). It often takes time to get to know someone and create a rapport that will enable them to open up and be honest—something that is vital for medical and emotional care. Without face-to-face interaction at the micro level, it is difficult to treat not only certain generations but those who might be seen and see themselves as minorities and to establish trust. It is difficult to open up to a faceless voice on the phone and this is more so when the faceless voice is unaware of the cultural nuances and tactile behaviour that characterise people's face-to-face interaction.

As the next interlocutor noted, many elderly first-generation Bangladeshi migrants choose to stay in Tower Hamlets:

> *There are a lot of elderly people living in Tower Hamlets and they are living by choice … because they wanted to live in a place where they can access essential services easily and without any fear and without disruption … A lot of elderly people want to live in Tower Hamlets because they can easily access religious activities … meaning mosque activities … They can afford and are able but they won't move out of the area because they are so used to and they wanted to be part of that … To some, they might not regard religious activities as essential but to our elderly generation, they regard religious activities as integral living or essential that they need to access and go to everyday.*

Many Bangladeshi Muslim elders in Tower Hamlets before the pandemic were used to the conveniences that the borough afforded. They are well integrated within their various social networks and knew the locations of shops, the various welfare services and the mosques.

Many younger Bangladeshi Muslims experienced the pandemic during lockdown differently, as a local government official explains:

> *Young people in Tower Hamlets now are very alive to what's happening in the world, especially because of social media … They get things on WhatsApp and a lot of the time I speak to young people and they send these reports to me … and young people have become very emotional in Tower Hamlets … They're engaged with what's happening.*

For them web-based technologies and social media platforms were a vital means of connecting with and participating in the world (Papaioannou, 2015). It appears that through connecting with each other and the wider world, digital communication has become an avenue for emotional outlets and a space where they are able to engage with and establish their positionalities in their own social networks and within the wider systems to which they belong.

7.5 Together Networks

During the pandemic, many things were not understood, and many tasks were done swiftly, sometimes without understanding the wider implications and the longer term consequences. Hence, it was crucial to have an effective meso level to facilitate access to care or food delivery, for instance. This is observed below:

> *People are very enterprising and find ways to do things within our communities that do support each other through adversity … so we're not really expecting the government to be able to make our lives better to be honest.*

Public trust was important for containing COVID (Liu et al., 2022), but, initially, at least, people put more trust in their own social networks than in the government, particularly those from certain ethnic minorities (Parsons & Wiggins, 2020). In terms of the different levels we have referred to earlier, at the macro level, the overarching care of the government for its citizens was managed through the vaccination campaign, for example, where greater trust in the government correlated with higher vaccine uptake (Thornton, 2022). However, when it came to dying and death, trust in the government was much weaker (see Chap. 6 in this volume). The high rates of mortality during 2020 created so much loss and mourning, which, often among Bangladeshis, is shared through local and transnational networks. People share memories, and relatives and friends come together for mutual support.

Mourning is a complex social and cultural process and the experiences that follow death are often multidimensional (Silverman et al., 2021). In the pandemic, however, it became a solitary gesture. Often, religious figures acted as guides and teachers to facilitate what was often an unfamiliar process for individuals who had lost loved ones because of the virus. Many people did not know the religious and cultural rites and practices that need to be followed in order to ensure a 'good death' (Islam, 2023; Gatrad, 1994). As one of our interlocutors explained:

> *There were instances, as I'm sure you know, where the father passed away very suddenly and the child had never had to experience death in this way or deal with a dead body in this way, it was a first for the family … In Bangladesh or here in normal times, when someone passes away, everyone comes to the deceased's*

house and comforts the family but we had a family here where the children did not know what to do because their father was the first to die in this way, he had died in the hospital and they didn't know what to do or where to go … This is not somebody's daily routine and it was very sudden … People suffered immensely because of this…

Mourning together is part of Bangladeshi culture and people's networks provide crucial support at these times. Comfort is given in various ways, emotionally and physically. People often bring food to the deceased's family, make arrangements for their welfare and offer words of comfort; support is offered mostly by friends and family during this time (Spruyt, 1999). Before the pandemic, local social networks were crucial in helping the bereaved understand and partake in rituals as well as cope with bureaucratic issues since many Bangladeshi elders died in hospitals and hospices (Gardner, 1998). During the pandemic lockdown, communal comfort was prohibited and the telephone became the key instrument which enabled people to collectively mourn. Local networks became crucial to helping Bangladeshis in Tower Hamlets negotiate with official NHS structures and other institutions involved in the process of death and dying, such as funeral services.

Care is a crucial factor in bringing people together. It relates to a sense of trust at the micro level through the operation of social interaction and social networks as well as at the macro level through hospitals, care homes and access to healthcare. During the pandemic, community health workers became important in building trust, especially with those who were vulnerable (Van den Bossche et al., 2022), and as we have already seen, Covid Champions played a key role as volunteers in promoting trust during the later period of the pandemic.

However, at the beginning of the pandemic, trust in official institutions such as hospitals was low because the NHS was unprepared and the impact on ethnic minorities and other marginal groups was particularly harsh:

There are lots and lots of stories coming out where people were being denied medical care and then having to experience … literally watching their loved ones die if they didn't receive adequate medical care … I think you definitely saw that in the first lockdown, where communities felt very, very marginalised and racism was in its height being displayed …

I did see that in the community, definitely … and it was harrowing … You go into hospital, you think you're gonna die; if you don't go into hospital you're gonna die … You just feel really powerless when you hear things like that and then you see families knowing this is what happened … Their father died because he was scared from both ways … and there were reports coming out at the time that if you go into hospital you're gonna die … So there were issues of trust just because of people's experience

When people experienced first-hand the complications the healthcare system faced because of the pandemic, trusting information about who was undergoing treatment, how good the treatment was and where people were undergoing treatment became very important for local residents. A lot depended on how social networks were integrated into wider networks and structures.

Beliefs about integration play a crucial part in how we understand our own positionalities in relation to the spaces we inhabit within the micro, meso and macro systems to which we belong. For Bangladeshis in Tower Hamlets, time was an important factor in determining how death was understood and the performance of certain rituals sometimes depended on how successful people were in accessing mainstream resources as well as the time they have taken in doing so. We see this issue discussed through a comparison between different ethnic minorities which draws on the discourse of community:

The performance of certain rituals sometimes depended on how successful people were in accessing mainstream resources. The Bangladeshi community are the longest Muslim community here so that they had longer to do the integration.

The degree of integration within particular communities also depended on individual choice and people's different reasons for settling in the locality:

It depends upon the person coming to Tower Hamlets if they want to integrate or not … It works both ways … If people want to be a part of a community, they can be a part of the community, if they don't want to be part of a community, they don't have to be … no-one's going to force it down their throats. [Integration] could mean anything really … I mean it depends on the individual … It could be a single person, they could be a person with a family and children, they could have extended family members living in the borough … they could be working in the borough … they could have friends already living in the borough … People come for different reasons and under different circumstances.

Moreover, the constant migration to and from London highlights connections people have not only within the city, but nationally and internationally as well:

> *London is a megacity, it is the most important city compared to other megacities like Bern, Paris or New York … London's connection is much wider compared to other cities … London cannot shut down … If we have severe destruction, we have to close our airport … What Australia have done, that is not possible for London because it is so connected with neighbouring countries, especially European and international countries as well.*

7.6 Issues Around Choice and Freedom

During the project, we spoke to many people who represented or came to represent different institutions and bodies in different ways. One of our interlocutors represented one of the borough's wards as a councillor and gave his opinion about how the government had found it difficult to curb citizens' freedoms over a long period of time (for a more general discussion, see Kraaijeveld, 2021; Vasilopoulos et al., 2023). The meeting took place during the summer of 2021 so he was looking at how the situation had improved and how people wanted a return to 'normality' and freedom from government restrictions on social interaction:

> *[The government/community now] are prepared … I think they are prepared with all the resources and I think they know what to do and people are a bit more prepared as well … If you tell them that this is quite serious, they'll stop going to the mosques or they'll stop going to the community places … During the last 3, 4, 6 months even, until last July, people have gone back to some sort of normality. So it's difficult always to take something away … especially to take someone's almost freedom away and tell them to just stay home and continuously do that.*

Sudden restrictions on the freedom of movement, then, impose a great burden on all levels of a system—how people interact with each other, how they cope with a sense of loss (of movement amongst other things), when they are not allowed to physically interact with each other.

Persuasion by the government was backed up by official restrictions as the following comment from a community development worker illustrates:

Some people behaved contrarily but that changed significantly when people came to hear they will be barred or they will be refused access to certain [places] ... For example, some people won't be able to travel until they have had both vaccinations. So those kinds of claims persuaded people to take up the vaccine quite extraordinarily from what they had already believed or thought of about the vaccine.

The combination of exhortation and regulations enabled the government to persuade most citizens to be vaccinated despite a certain degree of initial hesitancy due to a lack of trust in the government and official information (Halvorsrud et al., 2023) or people insisting that individual freedom (and thus freedom at a micro level) could not be curbed at the macro level. Gozgor (2022), for instance, has argued that people are able to trust their government if they perceive them to have the expertise, technical know-how and capacity to optimise public health.

However, some people continued to distrust the government and the health services even when they were training to enter the NHS like this respondent, who was a young, female university student:

I'm not taking [the booster.] I don't know a lot of young people that are ... I literally don't know anybody our age that took the booster ... but that's another thing because they're forcing healthcare professionals to go and take it, which is actually a violation to human rights ... You can't do that ... We took two vaccines, fair enough, but you're putting more stuff into our bodies which is made in less than a year, which is a bit crazy ... It's literally [an issue of] basic human rights ... You can't force them ... All health professionals, they're making them take the vaccine.

This argument against taking the booster vaccine links with our contention that there was little room for flexibility and elasticity within the overarching structural system. Our interlocutor asserted her right to choose not to be vaccinated drawing on information she has accessed through her own network. On the one hand, people were willing to be vaccinated because they trusted in official pronouncements about the vaccine's safety and its ability to protect people from infection. On the other hand, a significant minority were unconvinced and insisted that the freedom to choose was a fundamental pillar of human rights.

7.7 Some Final Remarks

We have explored here the complex interplay of macro, meso and micro levels through our engagement with Bangladeshi interlocutors in the London borough of Tower Hamlets during late 2021 and from the summer of 2022 until the end of that year. We have seen the enterprising and novel ways that Bangladeshis individually or collectively battled the pandemic. Social networks played a vital role in helping people to cope with and understand their own position within wider structural systems. We have also seen that Bangladeshi networks were flexible as people adapted to changing conditions and imperatives. Bangladeshis were affected by wider structural forces and responded to these in different ways depending on such factors as gender, socio-economic status and age, for example.

COVID-19 has taught us the value, amongst other things, of technology and social media platforms—it has allowed us to work at speed and has streamlined laborious aspects of work that might have previously been deemed as archaic. There are, however, issues with access to such devices and technologies. Socio-economic inequality and age are two key factors that can prevent some citizens from becoming 'netizens'. During the pandemic, these factors deeply affected people's access to information and played a significant role with regard to vaccine uptake and hesitancy. Social networks and connections with those on social media platforms proved to be vital nodes of information and influenced vaccine uptake, highlighting issues around trust and resistance to governmental structures, regulations and information.

As we have seen, people's understandings and memories are shared through their social networks and this plays a key role in the process of integration. During times of crisis, these local social networks provide a platform for comfort and support as well as much more meaning than unnamed, faceless, 'imagined' communities. They facilitate movement, elasticity and change to a certain extent within wider, more solid structures and, as we have seen, elasticity and choice have significant impacts on people's sense of wellbeing.

We are still learning about the importance of the meso level in understanding the complexities of local and wider social networks and integration, especially when speaking about how ordinary individuals experienced the pandemic. As we have seen in this chapter, the meso level becomes a crucial platform in the dialogue that needs to take place between the macro and the micro levels. If dialogue does not happen, people are unable to learn from each other and teach us more about how local social networks fit into—and perhaps adapt to—wider social systems.

References

Anderson, B. (2006). Imagined Communities. In B. Ashcroft, G. Griffiths, & H. Tiffin (Eds.), *The Post-Colonial Studies Reader* (2nd ed., pp. 123–125). Routledge.

Anthias, F. (2009). Translocational Belonging, Identity and Generation: Questions and Problems in Migration and Ethnic Studies. *Finnish Journal of Ethnicity and Migration, 4*(1), 6–15.

Baumann, G. (1999). *The Multicultural Riddle.* Routledge.

Beaunoyer, E., Dupéré, S., & Guitton, M. J. (2020). COVID-19 and Digital Inequalities: Reciprocal Impacts and Mitigation Strategies. *Computers in Human Behavior, 111*, 106424. https://doi.org/10.1016/j.chb.2020.106424

Bentley, G. (2020). Don't Blame the BAME: Ethnic and Structural Inequalities In Susceptibilities to COVID-19. *American Journal of Human Biology, 30*, e23478. https://doi.org/10.1002/ajhb.23478

Bergström, J., & Dekker, S. W. A. (2014). Bridging the Macro and the Micro by Considering the Meso: Reflections on the Fractal Nature of Resilience. *Ecology and Society, 19*(4), 22.

De', R., Pandey, N., & Pal, A. (2020). Impact of Digital Surge During Covid-19 Pandemic: A Viewpoint on Research and Practice. *International Journal of Information Management, 55*, 102171. https://doi.org/10.1016/j.ijinfomgt.2020.102171

Frink, D. D., Hall, A. T., Perryman, A. A., Ranft, A. L., Hochwarter, W. A., Ferris, G. R., & Todd Royle, M. (2008). Meso-level Theory of Accountability in Organizations. In J. J. Martocchio (Ed.), *Research in Personnel and Human Resources Management (Research in Personnel and Human Resources Management, Vol. 27)* (pp. 177–245). Emerald.

Gardner, K. (1998). Death, Burial and Bereavement Amongst Bengali Muslims in Tower Hamlets, East London. *Journal of Ethnic and Migration Studies, 24*(3), 507–521. https://doi.org/10.1080/1369183X.1998.9976647

Gatrad, A. R. (1994). Muslim Customs Surrounding Death, Bereavement, Postmortem Examinations, and Organ Transplants. *BMJ, 309*, 521. https://doi.org/10.1136/bmj.309.6953.521

Gilroy, P. (2006). Identity, Belonging and the Critique of Pure Sameness. In S. P. Hier & S.P. & Bolaria S. (Eds.), *Identity and Belonging: Rethinking Race and Ethnicity in Canadian Society* (pp. 117–135). Canadian Scholars.

Gozgor, G. (2022). Global Evidence on the Determinants of Public Trust in Governments during the COVID-19. *Applied Research Quality Life, 17*, 559–578. https://doi.org/10.1007/s11482-020-09902-6

Halvorsrud, K., Shand, J., Weil, L. G., Hutchings, A., Zuriaga, A., Satterthwaite, D., Yip, J. L. Y., Eshareturi, C., Billett, J., Hepworth, A., Dodhia, R., Schwartz, E. C., Penniston, R., Mordaunt, E., Bulmer, S., Barratt, H., Illingworth, J., Inskip, J., Bury, F., Jenkins, D., Mounier-Jack, S., & Raine, R. (2023). Tackling Barriers to COVID-19 Vaccine Uptake in London: A Mixed-methods Evaluation. *Journal of Public Health (Oxf), 45*(2), 393–401. https://doi.org/10.1093/pubmed/fdac038

Islam, F. (2023). Pandemic-induced Deathscapes: End-of-life, Funerary and Bereavement Challenges for British-Bangladeshi Muslims. *Social & Cultural Geography, 24*(3–4), 409–427. https://doi.org/10.1080/14649365.2022.2130416

Joy, M., McGagh, D., Jones, N., Liyanage, H., Sherlock, J., Parimalanathan, V., Akinyemi, O., van Vlymen, J., Howsam, G., Marshall, M., Hobbs, F. R., & de Lusignan, S. (2020). Reorganisation of Primary Care for Older Adults During COVID-19: A Cross-sectional Database Study in the UK. *British Journal of General Practice, 70*(697), e540–e547. https://doi.org/10.3399/bjgp20X710933

Kraaijeveld, S. R. (2021). COVID-19: Against a Lockdown Approach. *Asian Bioethics Review, 13*, 195–212. https://doi.org/10.1007/s41649-020-00154-y

Liu, J., Shahab, Y., & Hoque, H. (2022). Government Response Measures and Public Trust during the COVID-19 Pandemic: Evidence from Around the World. *British Journal of Management, 33*, 571–602. https://doi.org/10.1111/1467-8551.12577

Nitschke, J. P., Forbes, P. A. G., Ali, N., Cutler, J., Apps, M. A. J., Lockwood, P. L., & Lamm, C. (2021). Resilience During Uncertainty? Greater Social Connectedness During COVID-19 Lockdown is Associated with Reduced Distress and Fatigue. *British Journal of Health Psychology, 26*(2), 553–569. https://doi.org/10.1111/bjhp.12485

Papaioannou, T. (2015). Digital Media and Youth Civic Practices: Strategies to Foster Online Participation. In M. Hadjimichael (Ed.), *Arts and Social Justice: The media connection* (pp. 17–32). Cambridge Scholars Publishing.

Parsons, S., & Wiggins, R. D. (2020). *Trust in Government and Others During the COVID-19 Pandemic. Initial Findings from the COVID-19 Survey in Five National Longitudinal Studies*. UCL Centre for Longitudinal Studies.

Poole, L., Ramasawmy, M., & Banerjee, A. (2021). Digital First During the COVID-19 Pandemic: Does Ethnicity Matter? *The Lancet, Public Health, 6*(9), e628–e630. https://doi.org/10.1016/S2468-2667(21)00186-9

Sampson, R. J. (1991). Linking the Micro- and Macrolevel Dimensions of Community Social Organization. *Social Forces, 70*(1), 43–64. https://doi.org/10.1093/sf/70.1.43

Serpa, S., & Ferreira, C. M. (2019). Micro, Meso and Macro Levels of Social Analysis. *International Journal of Social. Science Studies, 7*(3), 120–124. https://doi.org/10.11114/ijsss.v7i3.4223

Silverman, G. S., Baroiller, A., & Hemer, S. R. (2021). Culture and grief: Ethnographic perspectives on ritual, relationships and remembering. *Death Studies, 45*(1), 1–8. https://doi.org/10.1080/07481187.2020.1851885

Sommerlad, A., Marston, L., Huntley, J., Livingston, G., Lewis, G., Steptoe, A., & Fancourt, D. (2022). Social relationships and depression during the COVID-19 lockdown: Longitudinal analysis of the COVID-19 Social Study. *Psychological Medicine, 52*(15), 3381–3390. https://doi.org/10.1017/S0033291721000039

Spruyt, O. (1999). Community-based Palliative Care for Bangladeshi Patients in East London. *Accounts of Bereaved Carers. Palliative medicine, 13*(2), 119–129. https://doi.org/10.1191/026921699667569476

Thornton, J. (2022). Covid-19: Trust in Government and Other People Linked with Lower Infection Rate and Higher Vaccination Uptake. *British Medical Journal, 376*, o292. https://doi.org/10.1136/bmj.o292

Van den Bossche, D., Willems, S., & Decat, P. (2022). Understanding Trustful Relationships between Community Health Workers and Vulnerable Citizens during the COVID-19 Pandemic: A Realist Evaluation. *International Journal of Environmental Research and Public Health, 19*(5), 2496. https://doi.org/10.3390/ijerph19052496

Vasilopoulos, P., McAvay, H., Brouard, S., & Foucault, M. (2023). Emotions, Governmental Trust and Support for the Restriction of Civil Liberties During the Covid-19 Pandemic. *European Journal of Political Research, 62*, 422–442. https://doi.org/10.1111/1475-6765.12513

Werbner, P. (2005). The Translocation of Culture: 'Community Cohesion' and the Force of Multiculturalism in History. *The Sociological Review, 53*(4), 745–768. https://doi.org/10.1111/j.1467-954X.2005.00594.x

Werbner, P. (2010). Complex Diasporas. In K. Knott & S. McLoughlin (Eds.), *Diasporas: Concepts, Intersections, Identities.* Zed Books.

Wolhuter, C., & Jacobs, L. (2021). The COVID-19 pandemic: Streamlining or Capsizing the Global Higher Education Revolution. *Perspectives in Education, 39*(1), 291–303. https://doi.org/10.18820/2519593X/pie.v39.i1.18

CHAPTER 8

Good (Local) Governance and State Capacity: Continuity and Difference in Times of Pandemic and Beyond

Jörg Dürrschmidt

8.1 State Capacity and Migrant Integration: The Importance of the Local Level

The course of the Corona pandemic has shown clearly that the resilience of societies in times of crisis is largely dependent on the working relationship between the state and its citizens. The ability of the state to reach its resident population is as important as the active compliance of all its residents. One of the leading state theoreticians has aptly described this mode of governance, following from this relationship of mutual dependency, as 'state capacity' and argued that it comes most clearly to the fore in times of crisis (Fukuyama, 2013, 2020). Fukuyama argues in this regard that 'state capacity' always, but especially in times of a pandemic crisis, refers to the capacity of governments to enforce rules and deliver services across a

J. Dürrschmidt (✉)
Ludwigsburg University of Applied Sciences (HVF), Ludwigsburg, Germany
e-mail: joerg.duerrschmidt@hs-ludwigsburg.de

M. Caselli et al. (eds.), *Migrants' (Im)mobilities in Three European Urban Contexts*, Europe in a Global Context,
https://doi.org/10.1007/978-3-031-53773-8_8

variety of functions, levels, and communities. This capacity depends less on the body of law and more on trust in the professionalism of administrative staff, on the reliability of public institutions, and on convincing leadership. However, state capacity is of relational character since it also relies on the self-organizing capacity of the wider society.

The challenges posed towards state capacity during Covid-19 go far beyond measures of effective epidemiological management. Without exaggeration it could be argued that a pandemic is always also a litmus test of a society's democratic character as far as maintenance of social cohesion and consensus is concerned, not least through the reliable delivery of public services to the entire resident population (Fukuyama, 2020). In that respect it is an indispensable aspect of state capacity that the protective character of the rule of law and equal access to public services includes ethnic minority groups. 'The local last-mile delivery of routine services on a continuing basis' provides, in particular, the foundation of the 'social pact' that nourishes state capacity due to 'breadth of support in the general population' (Bardhan, 2022, pp. 72f., 93f.).

As we have already stated in our *Introduction*, there is good reason to investigate 'state capacity' in times of crisis at the local level. Speaking in conceptual terms, the shift of emphasis in the analysis of stateness from politics to policy implementation has led to an association of 'good governance' with high-quality provision of public services such as education or health care (Fukuyama, 2004, 2013). The idea of 'bureaucratic autonomy' (Fukuyama, 2013, pp. 6, 9f.) captures well the relative independence of street-level bureaucracy from political elites in the frontline delivery of public infrastructure. At the same times this autonomy 'does not exclude extensive collaboration with private sector or civil society organizations in service delivery' (ibid., p. 10f.). It is indeed at the municipal level where a great deal of public services for migrants are offered and where actual integration policy occurs. The municipal level has been strengthened by a 'local turn in migrant integration policies' across most Western European societies. And even if this has been accompanied by neo-assimilationist tendencies in national programmes of integration, national integration politics and local integration policies tend to remain 'two worlds apart' (Scholten & Penninx, 2016, pp. 98ff., 94).

The Corona pandemic has worked like a gigantic social experiment to further reveal the ambivalences of migrant integration at the local level. In a situation of local 'lockdown' the question of 'where did you turn to' or 'whom do you turn to' for orientation, assistance, and help raises the issue of institutional trust in public services and civil society organizations, guidance by communal and/or community leadership, self-reliance in ethnic networks, and/or on broader (trans)local solidarity. Moreover, a privatized 'solidarity of retreat' as an answer to a community-threatening unknown has reopened general questions of allochthone and autochthone belonging, single and divided loyalties, and deservingness within urban communities. Thus, during a pandemic crisis, it is at the municipal level where the balancing act between post-national solidarity on the basis of 'effective residence', on the one hand, and prioritization on the basis of legal 'citizenship', on the other hand, come to the fore most clearly (Triandafyllidou, 2022, p. 4f.). Migrants might experience this localized ambivalence even more so, since heightened mobility restrictions had undercut transnational embeddedness and a renationalized pandemic solidarity has exposed their precarious residential and citizen status.

The shift of analytic attention to the municipal level in order to understand the role of public administration during the pandemic, as part of a better understanding of state capacity proposed here, ties in with more recent tendencies in multi-level governance and migration research. More generally, cities have attracted new interest as sites of governance within a more fluid neo-liberal global order (Trounstine, 2009; Davies, 2014). This process of 'rescaling' has changed the position of cities both in relation to states and in transnational or global hierarchies of power. Migration research has in this context rediscovered the importance of the 'city scale' for 'migrant incorporation'. This terminology suggests the active participation of migration networks in the 'rescaling' of the city while, at the same time, the city itself is considered as a negotiable and heterogeneous social field (Glick Schiller & Çağlar, 2009). More recently, the notion of 'rescaling' has been linked to research on 'multi-level governance'. Here it has been argued that this particular mode of governance is not just prone to ambivalence and contradiction, but is also the source 'of remarkable innovation' (Ambrosini & Boccagni, 2015, p. 38). In order to further uncover this potential for innovation, attention is shifted to the 'horizontal dimension of MLG', referring to the multitude of private and civil society actors and institutions, including immigrant organizations themselves, that are involved in local (im)migration governance (Dimitriadis et al., 2021, pp. 251f., 262).

This turn towards the 'increasingly active role of the horizontal dimension of migration governance' (ibid., p. 254) offers not just a wider perspective on (multi-level) governance, but effectively draws attention to the 'dynamics *within* municipalities as well as power relations that shape negotiations over inclusion/exclusion [that] have so far been less discussed' (Homberger et al., 2022, p. 95). It is a question open for empirical investigation, if the 'proliferation of policy-making coalitions that only, in part, consits of representatives of the state', necessarily fosters a consistent 'urban culture of cooperation' that allows minority claims to be articulated and heard (Schönwälder, 2020, p. 1932ff.). The recent history of urban 'cultures of welcome' and 'cities of refuge' might indicate that local immigration policy remains a contested field where public and non-public actors 'interact, sometimes cooperating and in other cases conflicting'. The concept of 'battleground', therefore, seems just as appropriate for the horizontal dimension of (im)migration governance (Ambrosini, 2021, p. 379f.).

What instead is certain in this conceptual and analytical reframing of local state capacity is that despite some commonalities in the field of (im) migration policy, there is also a renewed appreciation of the 'variety of context- (and path-) dependent practices' in this policy field (Ambrosini & Boccagni, 2015). If there is indeed a 'national turn on local integration policy' as suggested by some observers (Emilsson, 2015, p. 2), this is not to be equated with homogenization of (im)migration policy at the municipal level. Instead, we would support the assumption that 'minor contextual differences', such as administrative structure, migration history, civil society tradition, and urban leadership, can make a difference in terms of local social cohesion in times of a pandemic (Vertovec, 2020, p. 24). It is to these contextual differences that we will now turn by drawing on the three local case studies introduced in Chaps. 2, 3, and 4.

8.2 Resilient Urban Culture of Cooperation: Stuttgart

Within our three case studies, Stuttgart lends itself to an exemplary investigation of the functioning of an 'urban culture of cooperation' in times of a crisis for various reasons. Germany belongs to those countries in Europe that admit to their local authorities a relatively strong position within the (nation) state structure. This means that the local level not only administers national and regional law but retains some autonomous functions, especially with regard to cultural and social life. At the same time, Stuttgart embodies in exemplary fashion the path-dependent tendency towards a 'proliferation of policy-making coalitions that only in part consist of representatives of the state' (Schönwälder, 2020; Giersig cited in Schönwälder, 2020, p. 1934).

Already in the aftermath of guest worker migration, Stuttgart's back then mayor, Manfred Rommel, described the city as a 'multicultural society'. Until now, and despite having different political orientations, his successors have continued a pragmatic integration policy that regards migration as a precondition for innovation and sustainable economic growth (Meier-Braun, 2009). Accordingly, a dense web of organizations representing migrant life in Stuttgart has emerged and is engaging in dialogue and participation with local politics. For instance, there is the 'Stuttgart Council of Religions', which was established in 2015 with a roll-on informal leadership. Between 2019 and 2021, a representative of *DITIB* (German abbreviation of Turkish-Islamic Union for Religious Affairs) served as head (coordinator) of this interreligious forum. The latter is symbolically important because the Turkish Muslim community has been the prime focus where integration politics and policy in Stuttgart are concerned. Overall, Stuttgart's integration policy could be described as following a sustainable pattern of 'integrationism' (Nieswand, 2021). It describes a frame of action and meaning that builds bridges between actors in politics, civil society, and everyday life by providing an ideology-like legitimation order around the moral hypergood of integration (see more detail in Chap. 3).

We have further investigated this 'urban culture of cooperation' within a Stuttgart borough where the Turkish community has a significant presence. Presence here does not primarily mean numbers, since it is a mixed neighbourhood and there are boroughs with a higher percentage of people with Turkish descent. It refers to the presence of a DITIB mosque whose regional catchment area makes the borough a hub of Turkish life in the Stuttgart metropolitan region. In the following I shall outline those elements of an 'urban culture of cooperation' based on 'integrationism' as they emerge from our interview material.

To start with, we found a functioning division of labour within the borough council leadership, based on a division of tasks and competencies but also coupled with a shared sense of commitment to matters of integration. While the head of the borough council[1] would mainly take over representative projects, her deputy would deal with the nitty-gritty of

[1] Literally in German: *Stadtbezirksvorsteherin*.

public administration, including migrant-related service delivery. Moreover, both can be sure that this commitment to integration matters is shared not only by their counterparts in the other Stuttgart boroughs but also by the city's leadership. As the head of the borough council explains:

> *So above all, I'm the face to the outside, the contact person to everyone. But there are topics, on which my deputy works, very competently, and takes care of parts that are related to actual administration, which is becoming more and more difficult and more and more complicated. But we don't need to be prompted as far as integration is concerned. Well, I think, now I'm also speaking as member of a large city administration, the subject of integration already permeates the entire administration. It is an important topic backed by the authority of the mayor.*

This is by no means a benign statement with regard to a better understanding of horizontal governance structures as outlined in the previous section. For it is often assumed that the crucial aspect in the horizontal dimension of migration and integration governance concerns the implementation barriers deriving from tensions between public and non-public actors or government and civil society actors (Ambrosini, 2021, p. 376f.). Less attention is given to the fact that an 'inclusive approach' to migrant incorporation within a municipality is a matter of 'cooperation between the departments' and that it is, indeed, 'a policy adopted by the city council as a whole' rather than a token policy by one or two of its departments (Homberger et al., 2022, pp. 99, 104).

Moreover, when the new research into the horizontal working of governance mentions 'a wider approach to governance' that most European local authorities are said to have developed (Ambrosini & Boccagni, 2015, p. 45), this seems also to imply that its representatives tend to develop a moral commitment to their task. Rather than pursuing a rational choice and rule by law-oriented mode of governance, we found evidence of strong emotional undertones in the borough council leadership's narrative on personal accountability. This ties in with Fukuyama's claim (2013, pp. 2, 12) that good governance in the realm of public administration can no longer simply follow the Weberian ideal of the 'rule-bound implementers' of decisions made elsewhere. Instead, Fukuyama continues, these 'highly educated professionals' will be 'guided by internal norms' as well. The deputy council leader refers to this in a somewhat matter of fact way by saying:

Yes, of course, there was always this 'I want this' in play as well. I would say that it just came along with the task.

While the borough council leader is almost philosophical about this:

Yes, you have to be there with the heart, even in such a dry environment as public administration [laughs]. Well, in any case, I receive feed back from people of all kinds rather often that one can tell that I enjoy doing it or speak from the heart, and then that's how it is.

This emotional and personalized attitude to job and role is useful when liaising with the local Turkish community, especially the representatives of the DITIB mosque association. The borough council leader describes what she labels as 'personal address' in more detail as follows:

I don't email, I usually go there. It's usually a face-to-face meeting or a phone call now and then. It usually goes through Mr. I. [DITIB representative] and me, or Mr. C., the chairman of the mosque association here, with whom I have a very good rapport. I would say I am completely familiar with them, and if something is going on or something, it always works.

The DITIB representative comments in a similar tone and terms:

Human effort is an important part of it, both on our side as well as the government side. The paths are known, the structures are there, you just have to make the effort. To simply approach one another is the name of the game, and you just have to, well have the heart to do it.

This kind of interpersonal mode of familiarizing communication is made possible by the room for manoeuvre opened up by the steady devolution of immigration policy to the local level. In this respect the often emphasized 'discretionary power' of the street-level bureaucrat is directed towards showing respect and social recognition towards partners in integration matters (Dimitriadis et al., 2021, p. 257; Homberger et al., 2022, p. 107f.). The borough council leader testifies to the relative autonomy of the horizontal dimension of local governance:

We are not so tightly integrated within the administrative hierarchy. An essential part of our work is also community work and citizens participation. And there we do have a lot of leeway. And you have to, you can use it.

When pressed to characterize the relationship of trust and coordination between local authority and migrant association as either institutional or personal trust, both sides refuse such a polarization. The council leader comments: 'Because it is an area of sensitive change, you have to gain trust again and again, and having the flair for it', while the DITIB representative responded: 'That is, ehm, a two-sided and well-trodden path that we walk again and again'. Perhaps what we find here can best be described as *patterned trust*. By this we mean a mode of trust that emerges from a myriad of small-scale acts of trustful coordination without evolving into a fixed institutional structure, such as an additional advisory committee that meets at regular intervals. Patterned trust could perhaps further be grasped by reference to the almost forgotten concept of 'fiduciary attitude' (Vaitkus, 1991; James, 1992). This concept describes the pre-predicative Corona that surrounds active trust in terms of 'readiness to be open to believe in the other', based on three further elements: consignment to milieu-specific, taken-for-granted assumptions in everyday life; commitment to a shared task; and an element of faith in the future based rather on shared values than short-term interests (James, 1992, p. 284).

It could be argued that it is trust patterns like this 'that undergird local social contracts', which tend to unfold their potential via 'a better utilization of local information, ingenuity and initiative, particularly in the targeting and implementation of public projects' (Bardhan, 2022, p. 39). In the Stuttgart borough under investigation, the long-term commitment of the mosque association and borough council leadership towards the project of a new representative mosque, seen by both parties as a cultural asset for local society as a whole, could serve as an illustration. Yet the cooperation during a life-threatening crisis based on an unwavering commitment to social cohesion and an inclusive approach to migrant incorporation particularly testifies to the positive efficacy which 'integration' as a social value can unfold. This is especially the case when it undergirds alliances between state and non-state actors in order to enhance institutional capacities of local governance. We might recall here the effort undertaken by the local mosque community to channel government information towards not easily accessible milieus within the migrant community, the carrying through of Corona-related rules and regulations, the organization of solidarity networks reaching within and beyond the Turkish community, as well as providing the venue and logistics for a test centre and a vaccination campaign (see also Chap. 3). There is no pun intended when the borough council deputy declares: 'Well, they solved that in a very *unbureaucratic* way, and that worked well'.

However, this microanalysis of a resilient 'urban culture of cooperation' based on a horizontal extension of governance actors would not be complete without taking local civil society actors into account. Civil society actors are said to have pushed towards more inclusive policies not just by expanding access to government services such as health care but also by taking on the role of intermediaries and gatekeepers between migrant communities and local authorities (Homberger et al., 2022, p. 105f.; Dimitriadis, p. 257ff.). In the Stuttgart borough which served as our case study, this role of social broker is taken on by a local pharmacist. Her business is a hub of local everyday life and her customers come from all walks of life. Due to a generation-old tradition the pharmacy also serves as an anchor of local collective consciousness. Long before the pandemic the pharmacist started a lecture series for local residents where health issues were discussed by invited experts. Her medium-sized business is also a local employer, with a considerable part of her employees having a Muslim cultural background.

She and others regard her pharmacy as a living model of successful integration via work and civic education, for instance when she negotiates with her Muslim employees the appropriateness of wearing a headscarf according to both cultural sensitivities and work-related practicalities (sales vs. backstage work). She keeps out of party politics but perhaps due to this neutrality she is well connected with the local administration. During the pandemic her pharmacy became a centre of health information campaigning and vaccination. In a rather self-confident manner she describes her position in the middle of things:

> *I'm a local business woman, and I'm simply neutral politically. I'm not doing the local administration a favour—no, not like that. But the Health Department once said 'We couldn't have done all that without you'. I am well-connected, so it was enough for them to call and say: 'If anyone can do it [an ad hoc vaccination campaign], it's you'. So that's all I need. I know that I have access to it [local administration], if I have something, I can call. I don't do that often, but ....*

Overall, this tiny fragment of 'urban culture of cooperation' deserves the somewhat enthusiastic metaphoric description provided by the borough council deputy: 'one cog is meshing with another'. However, this sounds almost too mechanical for the negotiated and also somewhat contingent way of 'horizontal' (im)migration governance' in times of a pandemic crisis. 'Smooth cooperation', as suggested by the relevant literature (Homberger et al., 2022, p. 102), seems more fitting.

8.3 Urban Culture of Cooperation as a Battleground: Stuttgart

If now, according to our 'sociological forensic' approach (Inglis, 2010), we interpret the microcosm of horizontal (im)migration governance as a latent 'battleground' (Ambrosini, 2021), we can see rifts emerging in the portrait of a 'smooth cooperation'.

First of all, the paradigm of 'integrationism', prevailing within the borough council's leadership, is by no means coherent but it does enable somewhat contradictory discourses to be bridged. Most notably we can notice an oscillation between two strategies. One involves an inclusive 'humanitarianism' (Nieswand, 2021, p. 86) that overlooks social disparities and cultural difference for the common good of the community in general and legitimizes an all-embracing space of solidarity during the pandemic, in particular. The other involves an 'essentializing moral othering' (ibid., p. 81) based on emphasizing particular aspects of migrant lifestyles. Often the former is used when legitimizing measures of inclusive biopolitical governmentality directed also at migrant populations. It is exactly in this vein that the council leader argues:

> *The vaccination campaign went really well, and sometimes I think we worry too much what separates us, even though we are all just humans. And people with migration background are moved exactly by the same issues as we are—like, how do I get my family through the pandemic?*

However, when long-term issues of integration—for instance, immigrant settlement patterns—are brought into the equation, particular forms of behaviour are essentialized into a group-related alterity with almost civilizational scope. Along this line the deputy explains the reasons for the higher impact of Covid-19 in Stuttgart's neighbourhoods with an above-average percentage of non-EU migrants:

> *And, of course, they are indeed to be found in cramped living conditions, where the families ... are living on top of each other very closely. And, of course, the*

fact that our foreign fellow citizens have a completely different understanding of family and solidarity than we do, also makes a difference.

Thus, while the discourse of inclusive 'humanitarianism' attempts the 'moral rehabilitation of stigmatized identities' (Nieswand, 2021, p. 77) through an emphasis on 'effective membership' and insisting on inclusive 'spaces of solidarity' (Triandafyllidou, 2022), the discourse of moralizing 'essentialism' revitalizes exactly this very stigmatization of heteronormative lifestyles in order to maintain what could be called 'hierarchical binaries' between 'them' and 'us' (Lewicki, 2018, p. 506f.). This indicates deep-seated ambivalences felt with regard to migrant population of Turkish background. Those, who are fully embraced as part of humanity, are at the same time considered with some reservations as far as their full trustworthiness in a situation of crisis is concerned. The borough council leader recalls:

Well, there isn't any evidence of a mosque-related break out of Covid-19 infection. I think people have held back a lot during that time, even though it was also an important time for them, with Ramadan and all that, and time for meeting with friends and socializing. So, they held back and just celebrated privately, as we did too. Well, I found that really remarkable, because there certainly were fears in that respect, and from my point of view, they have not come true.

It could be argued that 'hierarchical binaries' are part of 'a typical governmental technique' in post-migration societies called 'civic stratification' (Dimitriadis et al., 2021, p. 253). It organizes people into categories along a system of legal rights and social benefits with an underlying sense of 'deservingness'. It is a bordering practice attached to the 'moral hypergood of integration' that maintains and at the same time bridges the difference between long-term residents and migrant newcomers as well as between good and bad migrants (Nieswand, 2021, pp. 82, 87, 90). It seems evident that this bordering practice can turn into a 'battlefield' where not only entitlements are being negotiated but also civic values and questions of rightful belonging. It has also been argued that it is likely to be civil society actors that are actively pushing this agenda into a certain direction, thereby attempting to influence street-level bureaucrats into a certain direction (Homberger et al., 2022, p. 103).

In our case study it is the same pharmacist that initially saw herself as an active social broker of 'smooth cooperation' during the pandemic, who now throws down the gauntlet, initially towards Muslim migrants but then also to state authorities. Generalizing, but supported by lived evidence from people working for her in the pharmacy, she maintains:

> *Yes, it was all so uncoordinated. Yes, of course, there was no good cooperation because of the whole pandemic. The migrants are with us and are ultimately guests in the country. That is my understanding. So, when I go somewhere today and ultimately, I am a guest in the country. I don't think people see it that way anymore. People think they make their own laws. I had a lot of problems saying [to my staff] that it's a pandemic, it's not just a feeling, but that one should really take it seriously from a scientific point of view and not have the feeling that: 'Oh, it's not like that' and all the, what slander propaganda there was. I know many who didn't get vaccinated. Especially with our Muslim migrants, there was a kind of blocking, conspiracy theories and all that. That hurts. If you don't get through there because there is another intention, whatever.*

When she eventually takes one of her employees to court for violating vaccination and testing regulations, she feels let down by the state in the face of a rather Solomonic court decision, which leads to her more or less directly questioning state capacity in its scope and intention:

> *But I didn't dismiss her because she'd been absent, but because she violated German law, against the instructions from above and then against my instructions, which I had put into context, and that's where it ends for me. That's when I start thinking: 'Is the state that weak, or what's happening in our country? Who is being protected? Am I protected as a citizen or only looked at when I open my mouth?' That's what I'm thinking more and more, and that is in fact troubling me.*

An initial reading of this strong statement by what most people in the local community concerned would regard as a charismatic civil society activist could find it highly 'self-righteous', following McCluskey (2019). While she sees it as her moral duty to provide humanitarian help to all deserving migrants, she also radically challenges their status of belonging as soon as they depart from expected behavioural patterns and moral expectations. Perhaps one could also refer here to the ambiguities of a 'subversive humanitarianism' that wants to be inclusive due to the vulnerability of the migrant but at the same times excludes due to doubts concerning the moral deservingness of this migrant (Vandevoordt and Verschraegen cit. in Ambrosini, 2021, p. 379).

However, it seems that what is really opened up here in the wake of the Corona pandemic is the contested field of 'moral citizenship' (van Campenhout & van Houtum, 2021, p. 10). This has become an issue in German society especially since obtaining formal or legal German citizenship has been successively liberalized from 1990 (Lewicki, 2018, p. 505f.; Schönwälder & Triadafilopoulos, 2012). Righteous or not, civil society, here exemplified by the pharmacist, might see itself especially in times of a pandemic crisis as the guardian of 'civic values':

> *And more often I then think to myself: 'No, it's not like that, we are a free country here, we have worked hard for this and for me this Basic Law[2] is something very valuable'. And I tell you quite frankly, the dignity of the human being is paramount. Equal rights for men and women are in the same place. And freedom of religion is granted, but it doesn't take precedence over equality between men and women.*

In Germany the public discussion on deservedness in relation to 'moral' and 'formal' citizenship has centred on the Turkish population, since they were the ones making most use of the naturalization option offered by the citizenship law reforms introduced since 1999. In contrast to the 'elite migrants', who possessed an EU affiliation, Turks in Germany also felt that their ethnicity was the most 'symbolic obstacle' to their incorporation via citizenship. This implies that the act of legally obtaining citizenship was tainted by the widespread suspicion about their ability and willingness to genuinely accept liberal norms and 'German values', whatever that might mean in detail (Schönwälder & Triadafilopoulos, 2012, pp. 58f., 62).

However, should all this play a role in governance at the local level, particularly during a pandemic? If, through the lens of 'sociological forensics', we consider the urban culture of cooperation as a 'battlefield' from the perspective of the Turkish community, we see initially that the discourse of abstract 'humanitarianism' in the face of a pandemic is shared with the local council leadership, even with some undertones of a global 'risk society'. As the DITIB representative claims:

[2] German Constitution.

I think we are all affected by it. It does not only apply to the Turkish community or any communities, but, um, from the corona we, as a multi-society, multicultural society or society as a whole, um, humanity on earth, um, are all affected by it.

Accordingly, the horizontal alliance built with the local council in order to fight the pandemic via enhanced institutional capacity looks unwavering:

We are, accordingly, always available insofar as we are able to do something. And self-initiative also plays a major role. As a mosque association, we have always been following it for every last change, accordingly, and have also passed that along into our communities.

However, on closer inspection this alliance is not so united. On the one hand, when the DITIB representative later on says: 'We always did more than required by law in order to protect our community', one can detect a sense of fear, not purely related to epidemic developments, but deriving from the latent fear of cultural stigmatization due to non-compliance. On the other hand, there is a clear sense of a growing awareness by the DITIB mosque community of its political efficacy. This awareness eventually amounts to a clear challenge to the power hierarchy within the horizontal governance arrangement:

Of course, it's easier in a trustful cooperation: it is a team work, nothing else. You can also compare it with some sports where two are driving in a rally—a co-pilot and a pilot, one who actually just steers. … I don't want to make light of it now [chuckles], and the co-pilot, um, he actually tells him what the route is, what kind of steering he is supposed to do. … And, um, we as mosque association have this bridge function, um, so that we are much better able to reach the individual communities, um, that the authorities are unable to reach, or that [state] institutions are unable to reach.

Even if presented in a light-hearted metaphorical manner, one can sense that there is more at stake here than implementing barriers to Covid-19 measures. And so, when pressed on this issue, both sides reveal that indeed there are things that separate them, which the shared discourse of 'human itarianism', however, tends to gloss over. And, again not surprisingly, these issues evolve around civic values. The council leader claims from the state authority side:

We have already mentioned Turkey before and there it seems important to me to work on the issue of women even better. Because there I gather from my daily professional life, uh, [that] there is still more to be done, without now wanting to somehow, uh, overshadow the success and the activities of, uh, many active Turkish women there, but there is still room for improvement. I am very sure of that.

The other side perceives these value-related approaches as part of a prevailing societal undercurrent of Islamophobia (Foroutan, 2013; Lewicki, 2018) that particularly surfaces in times of crisis, such as the Covid-19 pandemic. Here notably the ill-timed and ill-placed iteration of the then Federal Minister of Health, basically saying that the intensive care units at the peak of the Covid-19 pandemic were largely taken up by people from a migration background, galvanized a societal discourse that is widely shared in elite circles as well as in public opinion. The DITIB mosque community representative brands this as outright discrimination of heteronormative lifestyles:

We were the 'black sheep'. Although the concepts were changing, one time 'Turks', then 'Muslims' and then 'migrants', in this crisis we were the 'black sheep' again. That is, of course, the discriminating attitude hostile to Islam that was, um, expressed by this person. So, what I've been saying all along was, society is becoming more and more polarised, um, against Muslims, hostility to Islam, Islamophobia, group-related misanthropy, etc., those are the big issues that are currently interesting us in our society. And the task here is with government not to bring these minorities into an offside situation somehow.

This, besides indicating the ideological cleavages opening up underneath a pragmatic working alliance of local urban (im)migration governance, also shows that despite their acclaimed room of manoeuvre, these horizontal arrangements are nevertheless tied up in transnational and vertical contingencies (Homberger et al., 2022, p. 103). The local council for its part, and as a crucial level of a vertical multi-level governance system, has to keep a precarious balance between the 'neo-assimilationist' guidelines of integration policy around the principles of civic values and social cohesion as imposed from above, and a pragmatically maintained 'multiculturalist subtext' under the label of 'diversity management' at the level of communal public administration (Ambrosini & Boccagni, 2015, pp. 36, 42f.).

Its partner, the local DITIB mosque community, can in turn itself be regarded as a 'contested space' caught up in 'religeopolitics' (Öcal & Gökarıksel, 2022). While it is legally a civil society organization, and thereby subject to German law, at the same time it continues to have institutional ties to the Turkish state via the government body called the Directorate of Religious affairs, which is responsible for imam training, for example. Amidst claims made by either side, the DITIB mosque communities struggle to maintain a diasporic identity rather than being seen as transplant of the Turkish state or a tool of German neo-assimilationist policy.

8.4 Post-multiculturalism and the NHS as a Strong Institution: London

Looking across to London for the sake of further analytic contrasting, we have initially to acknowledge similarities. The Bangladeshis in London, especially in the borough of Tower Hamlets, are a settled ethnic minority. Accordingly, we found a dense web of civil society-based migrant institutions, mainly in the mode of trusts. These have a long tradition of helping to maintain Bangladeshi cultural life and heritage, but they also contribute to London's festival culture and cooperate with local government in matters of youth education and prevention policies. Crucial players within this web of cooperation, just as has been highlighted in the Stuttgart case, are the mosque associations. This long-standing pattern of cooperation has, next to the prevalent features of efficient local cooperation, also aspects of a battleground about integration policies. This perhaps even more so than is the case in Stuttgart, due to the sheer number and symbolic significance of Bangladeshi life and culture in the London borough of Tower Hamlets (see Chap. 2).

Nevertheless, this settled pattern of cooperation could be activated during the Corona pandemic for the emergency issues and tasks, which are familiar already from the Stuttgart section of the chapter: the organization of vaccination education campaigns for Bangladeshis, the pop-up vaccination facility organized by the East London Mosque, the organization of catch-up schooling and computer facilities during periods of home schooling, the transmission of government information in ethnic minority language, as well as the organization of everyday help for those in need, for example, via food banks, to name just the most obvious aspects of the ethnic minority-based infrastructure of self-help.

However, there are two distinct features in the London case to which we wish to draw attention in order to get a more sophisticated picture of good local governance during the Corona crisis. These are the incomplete transition from multiculturalism to 'post-multiculturalism' (Vertovec, 2019) and the role played by the NHS as an 'anchor institution' within the neo-liberal reframing of health care (The Health Foundation, 2019).

With regard to the first aspect it can be maintained that London particularly testifies to the above-mentioned claim by Ambrosini and Boccagni (2015, p. 49) that despite neo-assimilationist national rhetoric there continues to be 'a variable, if generally significant persistence of multiculturalism' in European cities due to a path-dependent and pragmatic approach towards integration at the local level. With local integration policy largely left to the individual boroughs by the GLA (Greater London Authority), Tower Hamlets with its significant Bangladeshi population is a case in point. Official mainstreaming of local policy and public services followed the discourse of (local) 'community cohesion', yet this framework 'was sufficiently broad and flexible to accommodate local [multi-cultural] policy practices already in existence' (Scholten, 2016, p. 983f.). This implies a 'post-multicultural' situation where policies 'seek to have it both ways'—strengthening societal integration by improving opportunity for all, while, at the same time, continuing with culturally sensitive local policy and public service provision (Vertovec, 2019, p. 175).

Although this has not necessarily led to a more sustainable de-ethnicized dialogue between ethnic communities, it has helped to increase socio-economic mobility for some and thereby increased status differences within ethnic minority groups (ibid., pp. 172, 175). Long-term observers of the Bangladeshis community in Tower Hamlets have referred to a noticeable 'hour-glass' phenomenon (Eade & Garbin, 2002, p. 139, 2006, p. 182) where many remain in the lower levels of the service sector, while some of the second- and third-generation Bangladeshis have pushed themselves successfully through higher education and are now located in the elite service sector of the global city. There are a considerable number of Bangladeshis now working for local government, but also the National Health Service (NHS) has become a major employer.

Accordingly, in our interviews in Tower Hamlets we found less of the 'ethos of mixing' commonly assumed as the 'natural' grammar of interaction in a place of 'superdiversity' such as London (Wessendorf, 2013). As one of our everyday interlocutors described her perception of life in the Tower Hamlets neighbourhood:

Yes, it's very multicultural, there are lots of Asians here, I think there are about 60% Muslims here in the borough. The neighbourhood is comfortable, I like it here. We have friends who live in other boroughs … but Bangladeshis will want to live near other Bangladeshis. People want by and large to live near their own community, and for my friends and relatives, we all live near the Bangladeshi community, so our experiences are similar.

A trustee working for one of the Bangladeshi cultural heritage foundations in London looks at long-term developments and the impact of the Covid-19 crisis in a more reflexive manner, but still supports the meanings implied by the previous interlocutor:

I haven't noticed any changes. I think people are still living within their own bubble or within their own … perhaps segregated is too strong a word … but perhaps within their own communities. So, the Bengalis have their own networks of Bengalis … the white communities have their own networks. Where I think people might have come together more perhaps is in the foodbanks where people … poor people but of different nationalities and or faith communities would come together to collect food. … So that's one place where you would probably get mingling or interaction of different communities and the other places would probably be the Covid test centres and the vaccination places. … Other than that, I think communities stuck to their own networks.

While it is perhaps not surprising that people live or perceive their lives as located within a rather closed everyday milieu, we found the same strong sense of community-belonging also in interviews with representatives of the elite within the 'hour-glass'. A borough councillor and an NHS doctor both refer to the Bangladeshi community as 'my own community'. The NHS doctor gives a sense of the persistent gap between the Bangladeshi community and mainstream health care in a situation of 'post-multiculturalism' when he states:

I think the main message I said to people from the Bangladeshi community was: 'Don't forget before I'm a doctor, I'm your friend or another Bangladeshi or a person from the community. … I grew up here, I went to school here, I come from the community.' You can associate yourself with those places and I tried to build trust in something mutual from the get-go before I went into the medicine, because often people, they feel they get ignored when they come into some sort of interaction with someone who doesn't speak the same language as them.

This statement needs some further contextualization concerning the role of the NHS with regard to integration and health policies. Within the NHS doctors like the interlocutor have become an important face of the NHS. While in terms of sheer numbers they make up part of the categorization 'Asian', which next to 'whites' (50%) account for 32% of the HCHS (Hospital and Community Health Service) doctors working for the NHS,[3] their symbolic significance goes beyond that. In June 2020 a female British Bangladeshi general practitioner (GP) was part of a billboard campaign that portrait NHS staff to celebrate the NHS' 72nd anniversary and honour the role of frontline staff at the onset of the Covid-19 pandemic.[4] More generally they are perceived and perceive themselves as a 'model minority within hospitals' and as 'superhero immigrants' who have made good use of educational attainment in order to improve social status and cultural integration. At the same time, these model immigrants experience discriminatory stereotyping against the patient population of their community with lower social status, as exemplified by the 'Mrs Bibi Syndrome'.[5] In the words of our interlocutor: 'Medical School was a way of acceptance, so that white middle class people have accepted me into their space'. And yet, when referring to 'ethnic minority doctors' also having the task 'to start protecting our own community', he also refers to the 'so-called Bibi syndrome, which talks about Bangladeshi women exaggerate their pain symptoms'.

In effect, our interlocutor finds himself in a position where next to his medical expertise his skills in translating cultural difference (between state institutions such as the NHS and Bangladeshi community) and social disparity (between his Bangladeshi patients and himself) are also in demand. In this he is by no means confined to medical tasks or the clinical side of his daily work as an A & E doctor (Accident & Emergency). In his regular 'outreach work' via the media as well as in schools and, most importantly, through the consultative bodies of the Bangladeshi community and the state alike, he attempts to narrow 'that disconnect between policy makers and the community'. Translating health policy during Covid-19 for both the community and the state makes him feel like a 'middleman between the two'.

[3] https://www.ethnicity-facts-figures.service.gov.uk [20.06.2023].

[4] https://www.southasiamonitor.org/societydiaspora/british-bangladeshi-doctor-becomes-face-nhs-it-marks-72nd-anniversary [20.06.2023].

[5] https://mediadiversified.org/2018/09/14/mrs-bibi-syndrome-the-medical-stereotype-undermining-elderly-asian-women/ [07.09.2022].

> *Because a lot of the people that I care about or that I want to serve are my friends and family and people that I have personal connections with … and so when I go to these meetings with government and policy makers and people who make the big decisions, it's a personal battle because I can see it from their point of view too.*

With regard to 'overcrowding' as a field of intersection between health policy and post-multicultural integration policy he draws on his own experience:

> *No policymaker can explain overcrowding to me because they've read it in a book or they've read it in a paper, but I've lived it, and so to say that we'll send people to hotels or we'll do this and that policy … it's not that easy mate. … It's not what you think it is because you've not lived it. It makes sense in your head that it's just an overcrowded house—we'll just create more space—but what about that family dynamic or that cultural dynamic or that cultural aspect of it that you don't understand? … Like, if my dad got Covid and then if I had to live in a separate house or a hotel … that's just not something I would do.*

The latent 'battlefield' (Ambrosini, 2021) described here that unfolded in the wake of the Covid-19 pandemic between an ethnic minority community and the state, between health policy and integration policy, between pandemic measurements and culturally sensitive health policy is intrinsic to the NHS as a state institution. As such, it has undergone a deep transformation over the last decades from a tax-financed health provider under state authority to a neo-liberal state institution. It describes itself as an 'anchor institution' with a broad understanding of 'good health' and 'with access to clinical care playing an important but more minor role' (Health Foundation, 2019, p. 6). It seeks to influence the health and wellbeing of the local populations through career opportunities, local procurement, and capital investment, as well as high environmental standards. In order to achieve the delivery of a health policy with additional 'social value' it seeks the collaboration of other local bodies (ibid., pp. 6f., 9) and this strategy is part of a long-term restructuring of the NHS starting in the 1970s. This restructuring saw the loss of 'clinical autonomy' in the sense of self-regulating medical professional autonomy and the development of a 'scientific-bureaucratic medicine' where external science experts set the benchmarks for best medical practice while context-insensitive bureaucratic rule oversees its application (Harrison & Ahmad, 2000, p. 138f.).

The effect of these 'corporatist relations with government' has been to forge 'a symbiotic relationship' between a health care institution and the state. This process might enhance the 'managerial capacity of the state', but whether it induces state capacity—a capacity that always also relies on state legitimacy—is doubtful (ibid., pp. 138, 141). Already at the peak of this restructuring of frontline health care delivery, the 'deprivileging of ethnic health concerns and racist definitions of their needs' was predicted as a result of neo-liberal 'health-care rationing' under the clever formulation of 'clinical governance' (ibid., p. 141f.).

In his discussion of good governance and state capacity Fukuyama (2004, p. 73) maintains that 'the degree of discretion that an organization grants to a subordinate division, branch, office, or individual, is amongst the most important institutional design decisions that can be made'. If one is to follow this claim then the degree of 'delegated discretion' is important for finding the right balance between efficiency and control, because 'delegated discretion' is important in order to mobilize the social capital of cultural norms and values for the benefit of an institution and its capacity to deliver the desired outcome. Furthermore, by their very nature these informal or cultural modes of institutional embeddedness cannot be formalized to the degree that formal rules can, because they are person-related and context-sensitive (ibid., pp. 44, 29f.).

Consequently, it could be argued that the changes within the NHS organizational structure amount to an 'authoritarian transition' (Fukuyama, 2004, p. 27). Thus, when the representative of a Bangladeshi heritage trust recalls 'a vacuum' that members of the community have felt during the pandemic, she does not only refer to the fact that at the height of the first lockdown 'people haven't been able to see their GPs, the people they trust most with their health'. The 'vacuum' carries more than the immediate meaning, since it describes a feeling of nausea caused by centrally permitted guidelines and regulations that had little resonance among those who had limited familiarity with English or Bangla. The formal guidelines and regulations felt like a sudden impingement on lifestyle and culture by an anonymous authority. The 'vacuum' not only left space for misinformation but also created distrust.

Indeed, we could argue that, unlike the Stuttgart scenario, the issue here is not so much misinformation, since in Tower Hamlets misinformation was countered by, *inter alia*, animation films in oral languages such as

Sylheti. What was different from the Stuttgart case was the lack of trust in a state institution that peaked during Covid-19 but had a longer history. As the British Bangladeshi NHS doctor points out:

> *I mean technically, it is a government thing—the NHS is a government thing—but up until the pandemic it was always seen as a safe haven [by the Bangladeshi community], but once it all started merging into one … blurred system, it was a lot more difficult for people to trust it.*

The Bangladeshi trustee, referenced before, takes up this discourse of distrust and relates it to the prevailing tensions between the state and marginalized communities:

> *People are going to try and survive this pandemic the best they can with the resources that they have by trying to support each other, I mean … (sighs) … people from the East End don't really look to the government to sort their lives out. … They haven't done historically and I don't think they do anyway. But people are very enterprising and find ways to do things within our communities that do support each other through adversity. … So we're not really expecting the government to be able to make our lives better to be honest.*

In such as situation of a yawning vacuum of trust it needs the effort of charismatic role models like the British Bangladeshi A & E doctor to close the 'disconnect between policymakers and the community'. This is in line with Fukuyama's contention that 'interpersonal leadership' is a crucial source of state capacity (Fukuyama, 2004, p. 80), especially during a pandemic emergency, when social trust and social learning are just as important as the technical infrastructure when it comes to frontline public service delivery (Fukuyama, 2020, p. 1, 8). Thus, what might at first sight look like a growing commitment by an individual is, in fact, the adoption of a charismatic leadership role during a crisis. As the A & E doctor recalls with regard to vaccination hesitancy:

> *When the vaccine was, um … recommended by MHRA [Medicines and Healthcare products Regulatory Agency] and was being rolled out, I was able to talk to my community leaders. I did a Q & A [questions & answers] with the Imam from the East London Mosque on BBC Asian Network in Bangla talking to people about the vaccine. … I did loads of media work all in Bangla just to help people understand that.*

Nevertheless, the eventual success of the vaccination campaign within London's Bangladeshi community was makeshift in character and depends on a structural readjustment of the relationship between the government and the Bangladeshi community in the post-Corona future:

> *I think I'd describe it as it's borrowed trust and it's facilitating trust rather than building trust. ... What I mean by that is that I haven't made people trust the government ... people trust me. ... People trusted me to take the vaccine or people trusted me or the Imam when we did the Q and A—those are the people they trusted. Building trust with the government's not going to be something they watched on YouTube or watched on the BBC Asian Network. Rather it's those other aspects of the public sector that people have to have a positive experience of—so the benefits system, the welfare system, social housing, the education system, those sorts of things.*

Moreover, this makeshift effort enhances state capacity through the dimension of 'strength' but not 'scope' (Fukuyama, 2004, p. 7). Put differently, the charismatic effort of a Bangladeshi NHS doctor finds its limits not just in the disconnect between policy-making and community, but also in the capillary structure of a post-multicultural society, where the borders between the communities are consciously guarded:

> *It had a huge impact when we did the first [vaccination] clinic in the East London Mosque and when we did the Q and A session, but I was able to do that because it was a Muslim Bengali doctor talking to a Muslim Bengali Imam ... and we had that relationship. Whereas I felt like if I did that with the Sikh community, it wouldn't be as authentic. ... I'd rather a Sikh doctor do that and if I could empower a Sikh doctor or empower a black doctor to talk to the black Churches and people can have that relationship there ... then that would be more meaningful and more authentic than ... because otherwise it would be pretty much the same as a white doctor [talking to them], the authenticity would be fabricated.*

8.5 Latent State Absenteeism Meets Induced Associationism: Milan

Shifting our attention across to Milan and the Peruvian migrants living there, a less structured picture emerges. Instead of an institutionalized culture of cooperation between the local state and migrant organizations or a capillary system of multiethnic gatekeeping, as found in the established relationships between state and settled migrant or ethnic minority groups in Stuttgart and London, here in a context of 'new migration' the pattern of local integration governance is still settling down. Accordingly, the Covid-19 pandemic revealed the fragile structure of a still fermenting relationship that is characterized by reluctant state engagement met by a comparatively unstructured activism by migrant and non-migrant civil society actors and networks.

This situation is largely due to two interrelated factors: a half-hearted devolution within the field of migration/integration governance and the semi-legal status of many Peruvian migrants in Milan. Like the rest of Europe, Italy has seen a 'local government turn' towards mainstreaming in integration policy since the beginning of the twenty-first century. This has involved a 'devolution of powers to the regions' while, in turn, 'relations with local authorities became more complex' due to a plethora of partly contradicting guidelines and funding structures. This has resulted in an integration policy 'characterized by a complex and contradictory structure' (Campomori & Caponio, 2016, pp. 1, 6f.). In Lombardy this has resulted in a bureaucratic structure which negotiated between a regional office for 'Immigration, Detention and Poverty', 'Local Health Units' that despite their name operated in a translocal field called 'social zones' and combined health and integration issues in their 'social service plans'. Local authorities were also left largely 'autonomous in deciding if and to what extent to consider immigration issues' in everyday local policy (ibid., p. 8f.).

This inclination towards devolution is inspired by the long-lasting denial of in-migration by the Italian state, even though it being a significant reality since the 1990s. Ad hoc regularization laws—the last one initiated during the pandemic in 2020—can be seen as the central state's 'mainstay of immigration policy'. It is crucially relevant for a region like Lombardy, where 'two out of three immigrants who are regular today have been irregular to various degree at some time during their stay in Italy', i.e. where the 'paperless' status 'is considered almost normal' (Ambrosini, 2013, p. 177).

As a sequence of interview statements with Peruvian migrants in Milan during the pandemic crisis indicates, the Italian state is perceived as an abstract entity that during the pandemic was largely absent in terms of a coping strategy and infrastructure, while at the same time leaving those in semi-legal status in legal limbo:

The state and institutions ... 'I would say did little for us, I would say that the state, how shall I put it, we mainly took it onto ourselves to help each other';

Public institutions .... 'I'd say the state did nothing, apart from giving information about the pandemic, but that was all confusing even for native Italian speakers';

I mean, people didn't get the answers they were looking for from the state, because the state for a moment left them a bit on the back burner; they no longer knew if their regularization was going on or if they could continue their application for citizenship; but obviously, it doesn't just depend on Milan, there was a bit of difficulty at all the levels, municipality, region.

This amounts to a governance paradox. While the decentralization of state power and discretion of public service delivery are intended to enhance the flexibility and capacity of sub-state governance based on context-sensitive knowledge and networking, here it leads to the alienation between state and (a certain segment of the) migrant populations. In short, while the principle of 'subsidiarity' should mean 'that government is closer and more visible to the people it is meant to serve' (Fukuyama, 2004, pp. 67, 70), here it leads to a state capacity void due to the ambivalent 'decoupling' between national und subnational layers of governance (Campomori & Caponio, 2016, p. 6).

Into this 'void left by weak institutional arrangements', a cluster of stakeholder and actors of different political weight and organizational power has moved and established 'a sort of micro-social, do-it yourself approach' concerning local integration policy (Ambrosini, 2013, p. 177). The Roman Catholic Church and its third-sector organizations, especially in Lombardy, have a long tradition of providing social services to the socially disadvantaged, which increasingly included migrants. These institutions also provide an arena for new migrant networks in search of a basic organizational infrastructure (Campomori & Caponio, 2016, p. 7; Caselli, 2010, p. 61). What the comparatively new arrivals such as the Peruvian migrants particularly appreciate is the fact that 'the church helps with the difficulties in daily life—it's not just a question of worship and faith'. Practical help in terms of dealing with Italian bureaucracy is also provided by the numerous joint ventures between migrant associations and trade unions (Caselli, 2013, p. 76), such as the CAFs (tax assistance centres). As suggested by their name, these offer assistance with tax returns and tax compliance but also with other issues related to labour contracts. Beyond these routine services, they also offer informed help with regard to resident permits, regularization papers, and access to financial support by the state, not least during the Covid-19 pandemic. While our interviewees stressed that the service profile offered by any CAF is roughly the same, those 'managed by Latinos, make a difference for Peruvians in difficulty, since obviously Latinos feel more at ease with another person who speaks their language and above all understands their problem right, understands their point of view as a migrant'.

Finally, as suggested in another context of civil society enforcement of migrant labourer's rights (Bada & Gleeson, 2023, pp. 154, 157), the devolution of integration policy must not forget the importance of transnational stakeholders who help migrants to find a local 'voice after exit'. For the Peruvians in Milan and elsewhere this is realized via the Peruvian Consulate. Although the Consulate has little impact upon on the realities of Peruvian life in Milan, Peruvian migrants acknowledge its surrogate political importance: 'The Consulate is like a Municipality, it carries out all your registry activities, from birth certificate to identity card and they consult the Peruvian community, as if they want to give its citizens a voice in the world'.

Around this pattern of *substituting subsidiarity* has evolved a 'induced associationism' that is typical for Milan migrant society and its Peruvian migrants, in particular (Caselli, 2013, p. 77). It reflects the clandestine situation of the typical Peruvian migrant, experiencing a 'subordinate integration' while working in the 'new economy of three-D tasks' (dirty, dangerous, demanding) (Ambrosini, 2013, p. 183). With many of them remain nomads after arrival, i.e. moving between temporary jobs, from bedsit to bedsit, and often uprooting their whole social milieu due to the live-in character of domestic care work, the attachment to one of the various associations often provides the only fixed point for a 'community' that is, in fact, a loose and widespread network of individual migration destinies. Accordingly, the Peruvian associations have been characterized as an 'extremely heterogenous universe' with 'strongly personalistic features' (Caselli, 2013, pp. 74, 76). While overlapping networks might ideally serve the everyday help and solidarity of these migrants, it is less well suited when it comes to developing a political voice, in general, and engaging in dialogue with public administration, in particular (ibid., p. 76f.). Unlike the situation in Stuttgart or the UK, where migrant associations and councils are part and parcel of integration policy consultation and implementation and have found themselves in an institutionalized dialogue with state authorities and public administration, the situation for

Milan is different. Peruvian associations there have neither been seriously considered as channels for policy implementation nor their 'leaders' been seen as serious partners in integration policy.

The pandemic has brought this lack of institutionalized consultation between local state and Peruvian migrant associations to attention. As the representative of one such Peruvian association self-critically remarks, the rather unstructured way of network-style migrant organization made itself felt with the onset of Covid-19: 'In my opinion, synergies were not enough channelled anyway. … The pandemic then has somehow blocked all the associative ferment because people can no longer meet.' In consequence, many of the Peruvian migrants in sanitary and care jobs found themselves isolated especially during the strict lockdown policy at the beginning of the pandemic that some observers saw as part of an 'inconsistent' and 'unprepared' pandemic policy which was constantly 'mov[ing] back and forth between a disciplinary and a security rationale' (Pellizzoni & Sena, 2021, pp. 61f., 75ff.). For the Peruvians in '3-D' jobs this involved a clandestine life-world which was surrounded by unclear and contradictory regulations. As the president of another Peruvian association recalls:

> *No, we have Peruvians who work in hospitals, right? And therefore, they precisely filtered all the information necessary for the community and their families. No, I think they have been cut off, but perhaps precisely because of the irregular situation. However, at the beginning of the pandemic all of us were very cautious—that is, all of us, I mean both Italians and Peruvians—and therefore we also knew that we could not get out, right? There was a curfew, there were always checks, there were fines and this alone was a deterrent for many non-regular migrants—the fact of putting one's foot outside the home. Just imagine that maybe someone goes to get a swab test, they ask you where are you from, what you do, and many other questions.*

Speaking as a long-time observer of local integration policy in Milan, a local representative of the Catholic Church maintains that the pandemic situation of the Peruvians in '3-D' jobs was a disaster waiting to happen, caused not least by political inactivity:

> *The state, well, the state didn't even see them [the Peruvians]. … I can say I expected this to happen, nothing new, meaning that theoretically as a class they are not so different from others, but in practice they are … because they are a weak class, which the state was especially unable to see, and this is very serious, as was the medical implications for all of those who didn't have an Italian*

health insurance card (illegal residents), because although it's true that if an immigrant goes to A&E (accident and emergency) he or she has a right to ad hoc assistance [that's to say that even as an illegal resident, the person is entitled to emergency assistance and is identified via the granting of a designated health insurance card/number] but if this isn't made clear people won't know, and this is serious lack of foresight, not just in their regards, but because these people (Peruvians) live in close contact people at risk. They work as baby sitters, cleaners and most of all carers, so they could have acted as powerful vectors for the virus.

That the state even at the local level could not 'see' the clandestine Peruvian migrant milieu can be read as a reminder about the governmental technique of 'civic stratification'. It is executed via the administration of differentiated access to rights and services especially at the frontline of public services, namely the municipality. Those immigrants at its margins with only 'weak agency' at their disposal are most likely to find themselves 'outside' the legal-administrative system altogether (Dimitriadis et al., 2021, p. 253f.; Ambrosini, 2021, p. 386f.).

The municipality emerges in these situations as an implementer of contradictory rationales of 'emergency governance' during Covid-19 (Dimitriadis et al., 2021, p. 258; Pellizzoni & Sena, 2021, p. 77). It kept mainstreaming public services that did not include any specific measures for migrant minorities, while at the same time implementing an all-embracing containment strategy that sought to reach the marginalized migrant population, in particular. As a representative of the Social Service Department of the municipality of Milan recalls:

So, in my opinion [on] the public services side, no—in the sense that even the shopping vouchers and all the measures made with the mechanisms of the calls had more or less the same rules as always, so there was no particular focus on migrant people. Maybe, the only issue on which in my opinion there have been many exceptions is that of health. Ok, so with respect to the topic of vaccines, so, that is, we went a bit in derogation from other things, because there the topic was how do we ensure that everyone gets vaccinated? Here we deal with the serious marginalization of the homeless but I know that they have organized vaccination campaigns also for non-regular people, because the emergency that has blown up outside is that there are many irregular people in the cities and that if there is a health emergency issue, you cannot pretend that they do not exist. Wasn't easy, because they didn't trust them and everything … because let's say those, who are regular here in Italy, faced it like the Italians: so that is: 'If I don't want to vaccinate, I cannot go to work'. But that was a choice within a system. Those who are outside ... are not interested in getting vaccinated because they have to work, you had no leverage to push them, to force them.

However, this attempt to bring systemic order into the complex 'battlefield' of local integration policy during a situation of pandemic emergency only serves to shift this battlefield from bodies of public administration and local state institutions into the social fabric of the private family household. In other words, it makes the conflictual life-world dynamics of this 'battlefield' not only 'more visible', but relocates it into an 'unexpected context' (Ambrosini, 2021, pp. 380, 389f.). This shift is illustrated powerfully by a Peruvian live-in care-taker:

Then when the situation changed [after the first lockdown], the Church reopened, some could not come anyway ... because the family where they work did not want that they would go to Mass, and the family where I work asked me too, although they had already done Covid, so they ... in a certain sense were more positive, but still the family didn't want me to go out, but I wanted to go to mass. ... I know what it means to be stuck without seeing anyone and just going to work, I know what it means living alone, being permanently without contacts.

The statement vehemently claims the right to express religious identity in the existentially challenging situation of the pandemic lockdown. It is also analytically noteworthy, because it can be seen as indicative of the general struggle by 'invisible' migrant minorities to regain 'visibility' in Italian society (Caselli, 2010, p. 69; Ambrosini, 2021, p. 387). This 'battle' does not exhaust itself in de facto access to public services that they are de jure entitled to, but extends towards 'their freedom to express their cultural identity' (Dimitriadis et al., 2021, pp. 259, 253f.). The minute everyday practice of going to Mass against the will of the employer, to which one is tied in existential need, can thus be seen as one of the 'indirect and implicit tactics' that challenge 'the onto-political divide between migrants and non-migrants' (Artero & Ambrosini, 2022, p. 212). We might add, to a certain extent also between legal and illegal migrants. It should thus come as no surprise then that the inside/outside pattern, highlighted in the sorting attempts by public administration discourse, was taken up as a trope in the assessment of the challenges that a post-pandemic society will face by the leader of a Milan Peruvian association:

This is the point when it comes to immigration. ... Immigrants who have been here for ten, twenty, thirty years ... even in five years, you somehow trigger yourself in the system, right? Either clandestinely, or formally, but you come to understand the dynamics of the society that welcomes you and you live, eat, sleep, every day. ... Somehow you live, right? So, you have to know how to give an answer to ensure that this 'somehow' can enter the legal circuit of this country, right?

In fact, the aspiration to enter the inner (legal) circle of the society de jure, of which one has already been part de facto, can be seen as part and parcel of what has been described as 'struggles for citizenship from below ... by the persons directly affected by restrictive migration policies' (Dimitriadis et al., 2021, p. 262). Even if, as in the example cited above, these practices of reclaiming visibility have no explicit political intention and are rather existential in character, any attempt to fight restrictions in order 'to move, stay, work, live and survive' can be regarded as 'imperceptible tactical politics' (Moulin and Thomaz cited in Ambrosini, 2021, p. 387), not least because they often galvanize into 'strategies to create visibility' that go beyond self-affirmation and eventually generate the symbolic and cultural capital needed to enter society as a citizen in the full meaning of the word (Ambrosini, 2021, p. 387f.).

'Immigrant volunteering' is considered to be one such practice by which self-affirmation and civil society engagement are usefully combined. The achievements associated with immigrant volunteering range from social (e.g. sociability) and technical (e.g. soft-ware) skills and a better understanding of the unwritten mores of the host society milieu to the build-up of bridging social capital (Ambrosini & Artero, 2023; Artero & Ambrosini, 2022). All this supposedly works best when immigrant activism is supported by 'native actors', such as the aforementioned cluster of 'organized solidarity', which has evolved within trade unions and the Catholic Church, since these affiliations are considered to enhance both numbers and synergies, as well as providing the bridgeheads into society proper (Ambrosini, 2021, p. 388). As a more recently arrived Peruvian migrant pointed out:

The church is important, it's a pillar ... for a newcomer it's fundamental. Going to a church means finding people. ... The church is a benchmark for all newcomers, essential to find and meet those who are <u>already within</u> society.

The actual workings of these milieus of 'informal learning' (Artero & Ambrosini, 2022, p. 206) are described in the following statement by the female chairman of a Peruvian volunteer initiative attached to a Catholic Church parish in Milan:

> *The logic is this, within solidarity groups we share and tell stories ... we share difficulties and successes, and everyone learns from the other, no one has the solution. Some professionals (health workers or social workers) can help occasionally. ... Once we meet on the theme of violence, once we meet for the integration of the migrant in the local reality, that is the various processes that the migrant faces, how to educate children in migration. We have a specific program on this. This is our logic, and in the pandemic period we have tried to do this with chats and online communications; we write to each other and share information through the chats about needs and requirements.*

Thus, in terms of facilitating the aspirations of a citizenship from below, it seems that 'society has preceded the state and its institutions' (Ambrosini, 2013, p. 178). There is a remarkable sense of civic responsibility prevailing within these 'solidarity groups' which is expressed through helping in the organizing of sessions with dentists and gynaecologists for undocumented migrants, as well as family nurseries and food banks for those in social and material need, and sustaining all of this, more or less, during the pandemic. However, this is precisely where commentators detect the inherent ambivalence involved in 'immigrant volunteering' with regard to the local 'battleground' of immigration governance. While on the one hand activities such as those mentioned above can be seen as a 'useful tool and marker of successful integration', they at least partly 'take over responsibilities that have previously been appointed to public institutions' (Ambrosini & Artero, 2023, p. 254). By assisting with paper work, immigrant 'volunteering guardians' (Dimitriadis et al., 2021, p. 259) tend to facilitate restrictive migration and integration policies 'by smoothing the bureaucratic process' (Artero & Ambrosini, 2022, p. 211). Finally, they can be seen as part of a 'subversive humanism' that compensates 'for failing government policies' by operating along moralizing subject categories of vulnerability and deservingness (Ambrosini, 2021, p. 379).

Therefore, the notion of a 'citizenship from below' is not unproblematic in this context of a 'shadow state' (Ambrosini & Artero, 2023, p. 252). While for some it is just another way of becoming drawn ideologically into a neo-liberal version of 'ethical citizenship', others see it as having the innovative potential of 'lived citizenship' (ibid., p. 254). The first perspective stresses 'the technology of self' that transforms the migrant individual into a 'good citizen', who develops the necessary capabilities needed for 'civic integration' into a neo-liberal society, such as self-reliance and readiness to deliver free contributions in exchange for societal belonging (ibid., p. 254; Artero & Ambrosini, 2022, p. 206). The second perspective emphasizes the performative potential of 'practical engagement with the social fabric', which gives new meaning to 'citizenship' as well as breaks open the legal and other boundaries between inside and outside modes of formal belonging (ibid., pp. 2f., 11). While theoretically it may be impossible to decide between the generative and the affirmative potential of 'citizenship from below', the notion of 'lived citizenship' carries the potential to 'prefigure the claim for a more radical cultural change' (Ambrosini & Artero, 2023, p. 259). As such, it might have potential for a concrete utopia of a post-pandemic society. This is at least what could be detected from the statement by the chairman of a Peruvian association, who is also one of the few local councillors in Milan of Peruvian origin:

> *I believe that it is important that, in a moment like that we find ourselves, following the pandemic, which has put a bit of a strain on everyone, where there are no differences in skin color or origin, because it has affected not only Italy but the whole world. Therefore, it has put everyone on an equal footing. So, I see this as a great opportunity, to be able to stand up, to be able to rebuild our socio-economic stability and perhaps, why not?, it can also be a lesson for everyone to break down prejudices even more, and make our diversity in our society today work. And therefore, at this point, at this moment, I believe that politics is called upon to read the pandemic in this way.*

8.6 Conclusion

It is a truism that despite a shared tendency towards devolution and the mainstreaming of public services across Western European cities, the national and regional pathways of migration policy and integration governance persist. Moreover, state power has become more complex and contradictory, especially at the local level of governance. The 'sociological forensics' (Inglis, 2010) attempted in this chapter has not attempted to produce a conventional collection of 'similarities and differences'. Rather its aim was to describe the inner working of these local complexities and detect some logic or pattern behind each city fragment with regard to its integration policy.

By way of a postmodern conclusion, we could draw on Fukuyama's (Fukuyama, 2004, p. 43) claim that 'public administration is necessarily more of an art than a science'. Despite all the attempts to formalize the knowledge of the field of Public Management, 'good solutions to public administration problems' remain largely context-sensitive and interpersonal in practice. This chapter has shown that this applies to the intersection of integration and pandemic policy at the local level. By way of a more scientifically conventional conclusion, we would argue that all three city fragments considered testify to the increasing importance of 'humble governance' (Annala et al., 2021), which describes a form of governance that is faced with the 'wicked problems' of the twenty-first century, such as global migration and climate change. Primarily 'humble governance' departs from its conventional sibling through a fundamental assumption: 'acknowledgement of the government's fallibility' (ibid., p. 7).

'Humble governance' is based on constant iteration and learning, considers stakeholder as partners in a trusting rather than a deal-based relationship, and aims at context-sensitive policy solutions and public services. This means that 'humble governance' is, in practice, 'experimental governance', since due to the obvious gridlock in the structure and culture of contemporary governance there is no tool box of fit-for-purpose solutions for dealing with complex contestations like the Covid-19 pandemic and its impact on migrant/immigrant communities.

References

Ambrosini, M. (2013). Immigration in Italy: Between Economic Acceptance and Political Rejection. *Journal of International Migration & Integration, 14*, 175–194.

Ambrosini, M. (2021). The Battleground of Asylum and Immigration Policies: A Conceptual Inquiry. *Ethnic and Racial Studies, 44*(3), 374–395.

Ambrosini, M., & Artero, M. (2023). Immigrant Volunteering: A Form of Citizenship from Below. *Voluntas, 34*, 252–262.

Ambrosini, M., & Boccagni, P. (2015). Urban Multiculturalism beyond the 'Backlash': New Discourses and Different Practices in Immigrant Policies across European Cities. *Journal of Intercultural Studies, 36*(1), 35–53.

Annala, M., Leppänen, J., Mertsola, S., & Sabel, C. F. (2021). *Humble Governance: How to Realize Ambitious Reforms Prudently*. Demos.

Artero, M., & Ambrosini, M. (2022). Citizenship Beyond the Normative Script: Young Immigrants Volunteering as a Practice of 'Citizenship from below'.

Citizenship Studies, 26(2), 203–220. https://doi.org/10.1080/13621025.2022.2053504
Bada, X., & Gleeson, S. (2023). *Scaling Migrant Worker Rights: How Advocates Collaborate and Contest State Power*. University of California Press.
Bardhan, P. (2022). *A World of Insecurity: Democratic Disenchantment in Rich and Poor Countries*. Harvard Univ. Press.
Campomori, F., & Caponio, T. (2016). Immigrant Integration Policymaking in Italy: Regional Policies in a Multi-Level Governance Perspective. *International Review of Administrative Sciences, 83*(2), 303–321.
Caselli, M. (2010). Integration, Participation, Identity: Immigrant Associations in the Province of Milan. *International Migration, 48*(2), 58–78.
Caselli, M. (2013). Immigrant Associations in Italy. In V. Cesareo (Ed.), *Migration: A Picture from Italy* (pp. 73–76). Milano.
Davies, J. (2014). Rethinking Urban Power and the Local State: Hegemony, Domination and Resistance in Neoliberal Cities. *Urban Studies, 51*(15), 3215–3232.
Dimitriadis, I., Hajer, M. H. J., Fontanari, E., & Ambrosini, M. (2021). Local "Battlegrounds". Relocating Multi-Level and Multi-Actor Governance of Immigration. *Revue Européenne des Migrations Internationales, 37*(1 & 2), 251–275.
Eade, J., & Garbin, D. (2002). Changing Narratives of Violence, Struggle and Resistance: Bangladeshis and the Competition for Resources in the Global City. *Oxford Development Studies, 30*(2), 137–149.
Eade, J., & Garbin, D. (2006). Competing Visions of Identity and Space: Bangladeshi Muslims in Britain. *Contemporary South Asia, 15*(2), 181–193.
Emilsson, H. (2015). A National Turn of Local Integration Policy: Multi-level Governance Dynamics in Denmark and Sweden. *Comparative Migration Studies, 3*(7), 1–16. https://doi.org/10.1186/s40878-015-0008-5
Foroutan, N. (2013). *Identity and (Muslim) Integration in Germany*. Migration Policy Institute.
Fukuyama, F. (2004). *State Building: Governance and World Order in the 21st Century*. Cornell Univ. Press.
Fukuyama, F. (2013). What is Governance? *Centre for Global Development Working Paper, 314*, 1–18.
Fukuyama, F. (2020, July/August). The Pandemic and Political Order: It Takes a State, *Foreign Affairs*, 1–9.
Glick Schiller, N., & Çağlar, A. (2009). Towards a Comparative Theory of Locality in Migration Studies: Migrant Incorporation and City Scale. *Journal of Ethnic and Migration Studies, 35*(2), 177–202.
Harrison, S., & Ahmad, W. I. U. (2000). Medical Autonomy and the UK State 1975 to 2025. *Sociology, 34*(1), 129–146.

Health Foundation. (2019). *Building Healthier Communities: The Role of the NHS as an Anchor Institution*. Health Foundation.

Homberger, A., Kirchhoff, M., Mallet-Garcia, M., Ataç, I., & Günter, S. (2022). Local Responses to Migrants with Precarious Legal Status: Negotiating Inclusive Practices in Cities Across Europe. *Zeitschrift für Migrationsforschung/ Journal of Migration Studies, 2*(2), 93–116.

Inglis, T. (2010). Sociological Forensics: Illuminating the Whole from the Particular. *Sociology, 44*(3), 507–522.

James, J. C. (1992). Review: How Is Society Possible? Intersubjectivity and the Fiduciary Attitude as Problems of the Social Group in Mead, Gurwitsch, and Schutz—by Steven Vaitkus. *Contemporary Sociology, 21*(2), 283–284.

Lewicki, A. (2018). Race, Islamophobia and the Politics of Citizenship in Post-unification Germany. *Patterns of Prejudice, 52*(5), 496–512.

McCluskey, E. (2019). *From Righteousness to Far Right: An Anthropological Rethinking of Critical Security Studies*. McGill-Queen's University Press.

Meier-Braun, K-H. (2009). Zuwanderung seit 30 Jahren als Chance und Bereicherung: die Integrationspolitik der Landeshauptstadt Stuttgart gilt bundesweit als vorbildlich. In: Gesemann, F. & Roth, R. (Hg.), *Lokale Integrationspolitik in der Einwanderungsgesellschaft: Migration und Integration als Herausforderung von Kommunen* (pp. 367–382). VS.

Nieswand, B. (2021). Konturen einer Moralsoziologie der Migrationsgesellschaft. *Zeitschrift für Migrationsforschung/Journal of Migration Research, 1*(1), 75–95.

Öcal, D. K., & Gökarıksel, B. (2022). Grounding Religious Geopolitics: The Everyday Counter-geopolitical Practices of Turkish Mosque Communities in Germany. *Geoforum, 129*, 151–160.

Pellizzoni, L., & Sena, B. (2021). Preparedness as Governmentality. Probing the Italian Management of the Covid-19 Emergency. *Sociologica, 15*(3), 61–83.

Scholten, P. (2016). Between National Models and Multi-Level-Decoupling: The Pursuit of Multi-Level-Governance in Dutch and UK Policies towards Migrant Incorporation. *Journal of International Migration & Integration, 17*, 973–944.

Scholten, P., & Penninx, R. (2016). The Multilevel Governance of Migration and Integration. In B. Garcés-Mascareñas & R. Penninx (Eds.), *Integration Processes and Policies in Europe* (pp. 91–108). Springer.

Schönwälder, K. (2020). Diversity and political practice. *Ethnic and Racial Studies, 43*(11), 1929–1941.

Schönwälder, K., & Triadafilopoulos, T. (2012). A Bridge or Barrier to Incorporation? Germany's 1999 Citizenship Reform in Critical Perspective. *German Politics & Society, 30*(1), 52–70.

Triandafyllidou, A. (2022). Spaces of Solidarity and Spaces of Exception: Migration and Membership During Pandemic Times. In A. Triandafyllidou (Ed.), *Migration and Pandemics* (IMISCOE Research Series) (pp. 3–21). Springer.

Trounstine, J. (2009). All Politics Is Local: The Reemergence of the Study of City Politics. *Perspectives, 7*(3), 611–618.

Vaitkus, S. (1991). *How Is Society Possible? Intersubjectivity and the Fiduciary Attitude as Problems of the Social Group in Mead, Gurwitsch, and Schutz.* Kluwer.

van Campenhout, G., & van Houtum, H. (2021). 'I am German when we win, but I am an immigrant when we lose'. Theorising on the deservedness of migrants in international football, using the case of Mesut Özil. *Sport in Society, 24*(11), 1924–1940.

Vertovec, S. (2019). Towards Post-multiculturalism? Changing Communities, Conditions and Contexts of Diversity. *International Social Science Journal, 68*(227/228), 167–178. (reprint).

Vertovec, S. (2020). Global Migration and the "Great Reshaping". *Max Planck Research, 3*, 20–25.

Wessendorf, S. (2013). Commonplace Diversity and the 'Ethos of Mixing': Perceptions of Difference in a London Neighbourhood. *Identities, 20*(4), 407–422.

CHAPTER 9

Conclusion: Towards a Sociological Understanding of Layered Resilience

Marco Caselli, Jörg Dürrschmidt, and John Eade

As we stated in the Introduction, the COVID-19 pandemic operates as an amplifier, but not a game changer in matters of integration and integration policy. It has in a rather experimental fashion revealed the basic tendencies of cohesion and exclusion which are prevalent in all modern societies that rely on migration. Thus, our answer to the research question of the book—where do people with a migration background turn to in times of crisis—cannot be answered in an either/or mode. The Archimedean point between 'state capacity' and the 'capacity to aspire' is in fact a fuzzy field

M. Caselli
Dipartimento di Sociologia, Università Cattolica del Sacro Cuore, Milano, Italy
e-mail: marco.caselli@unicatt.it

J. Dürrschmidt (✉)
Ludwigsburg University of Applied Sciences (HVF), Ludwigsburg, Germany
e-mail: joerg.duerrschmidt@hs-ludwigsburg.de

J. Eade
University of Roehampton, London, UK
e-mail: J.Eade@roehampton.ac.uk

M. Caselli et al. (eds.), *Migrants' (Im)mobilities in Three European Urban Contexts*, Europe in a Global Context,
https://doi.org/10.1007/978-3-031-53773-8_9

of institutional and personal interaction. It is our argument that the pandemic resilience of a local society unfolds as a layered capacity that straddles individuals, communities, institutions and values (Mu, 2021). Although contextual differences and the path dependency of each research site continue to have some significance during the pandemic, there are a number of generalizable insights.

Firstly, the meso level, where front line public administration and civil society tend to interact, needs to be seriously considered so that we do not pursue a binary division between the state and local residents, in general, and migrants, in particular. The intermediary role of the meso level is important for all citizens but is even more significant for those, whose distance from the state—due to linguistic and cultural factors—may be greater than others at the same socio-economic level. The difference between Stuttgart, Milan and London lies in the nature of these intermediate actors and their degree of formalization—not in the prevailing importance of this fuzzy middle where state capacity and the capacity to aspire meet.

Hartley and Jarvis (2020) have proposed the term 'community capacity' to capture this fuzzy field of resilience and to some extent this fits with our research that has shown the importance of organized collective action, which is structured around migrant organizations with local or religious affiliation. At the same time, we also encountered many forms of private and interpersonal arrangements of solidarity and support that would not fit a clear allocation in the social realm of 'community' or 'civil society' for that matter.

Secondly, we would argue that in order to overcome the barriers of interaction and understanding between local state and migrant communities, we need what has been in another context called 'the capacity to connect across difference' (Hochschild, 2018, p. 13). We have seen that layered resilience is not just about structures, institutions, groups and individuals, but also about the order of values carried and embedded in each. If resilience is to be more than mere survival in a situation of crisis, then a pandemic such as COVID-19 brings the layered priorities of society to the fore more clearly. In other words, the question of integration and social cohesion always involves the integrity of individuals, communities and (local) societies (Albrow, 2014). For research into migration and integration governance, this requires, besides the usual focus on social inequality and cultural disparities, more attention being paid to what could be called 'the normative space of resilience' (Ferrarello, 2021). This in our view is very important for a social science-based understanding of 'resilience'. It would require more investigation into the everyday capacity not just to adapt and adjust to difficulty in life, but also to resist detrimental circumstances and even to see resilience as a capacity '[to] transform adversity to opportunity' (Obrist et al., 2010, pp. 285, 287).

Thirdly, it is not just interpersonal empathy that is required in order to connect across difference and to work the middle ground of layered resilience. Indeed, the COVID-19 pandemic has revealed shortcomings in the information and communication circuits between state authorities and migrant communities. It is a truism that the COVID-19 pandemic was also an 'infodemic' with repercussions on the course of the pandemic itself (Charquero-Ballester et al., 2021). Usually infodemic refers to 'six types of misinformation' clustering around virus, vaccine, cure, politics and conspiracy. Yet, more importantly, research stresses that misinformation, like any information, is never simply an empty signifier but is embedded in emotion (ibid., p. 1,3). This means that emotive and value-driven transmission of information cannot be countered via more information designed to counter myths but needs to be aware of the cultural sensitivity of information.

Our research found intense and laudable attempts by state bodies to multi-channel information and to use social brokers like the Covid Champions when established technology failed to deliver information to the difficult-to-reach sections of the migrant population. However, we would maintain that it is not enough to push technological frontiers in order to be better equipped in this aspect of state capacity for the next pandemic. The cultural sensitivity of information and service delivery is just as important, especially amongst the public servants engaged in the final stage of delivery. This can mean awareness of the narratives that circulate about past occasions where medical trials have used ethnic minorities as 'guinea pigs' and how this can be related to an awareness of resistance among family-centred migrant milieus towards quarantine measures that separate the sick individual from family support. It can also involve an awareness of the importance of the migrant body as a marker of symbolic difference that affects an individual's readiness to offer this body for vaccination or other emergency-related state intervention.

A fourth point following on from this concerns the durability of the spaces of solidarity based on effective residence that emerged during the pandemic. By the time of writing this conclusion, it feels as if society is caught in the 'death reflex of normality', as Ulrich Beck (1995, p. 48f.)

once aptly called the eventual return to accustomed normalcy even if its anyway fragile structure has just been deeply shattered by successive hazards in 'risk society'. No one, it seems, wants to be reminded about the roughly two years of a 'new normal' under COVID-19 restrictions but also opportunity. It is important to recall the deep urge for reflexive narrative in our conversations with local government representatives as well as representatives of migrant organizations and ordinary migrants during the height of the pandemic. More important than the concrete topics raised in the interviews, e.g. the COVID-19 impact on family and gender, on relations between the generations, on transnational belonging or on the role of migrant advisory bodies, to name but a few, was the deep awareness that it needs a post-pandemic narrative engagement in order to secure and strengthen the social fabric of post-COVID-19 society. Indeed, to borrow from Appadurai and Robles-Anderson here (2023, p. 1f.): 'forgetting is a wish for normalcy to return'—'personal storytelling is expression against disappearance'.

Engaging in COVID-19 storytelling, therefore, might be a way of working through the pandemic as well as generating a narrative that suits a post-pandemic society that is also a post-migrant society. Its purpose, then, goes far beyond the mere overcoming of personal and societal trauma caused by COVID-19 and its aftermath, because any maintaining of stories, to borrow from Appadurai and Robles-Anderson here again, 'is a means of tending to the social by building public culture' (ibid.).

The suggestion of using narratives to stabilize 'solidarity's fragilities' ties in with the idea of narrative as a generalized democratic project as put forward by the French social historian, Pierre Rosanvallon, in his essay on the 'parliament of the invisible' (Rosanvallon, 2014), issued way before the COVID-19 pandemic. In this essay he addresses the shortcomings of a representative democracy in an era of post-economic social cleavages and increasing fragmentation or even fragmentation of life-styles. Through his concept of 'narrative democracy' he envisages a new form of representation. The permanent narrative exchange between state and society but also between the various sections of a fragmented society might initially seem like the celebration of 'individualized singularity' but Rosanvallon maintains that this project will rather go to the core of the deficits of conventional democracy. It will help to 'de-cipher society' as a whole in its organizing mechanisms, as well as giving a voice to the marginalized groups that fall outside the conventional political and media representation of social life (pp. 17, 19, 22f., 24–28).

This idea of a narrative re-shaping of liberal democracy is to be welcomed as a means of making mechanisms of inclusion and exclusion more visible, of giving impulse to the societal imagination of a shared 'good life', and even enhances the sense of belonging amongst the marginalized. However, and this is the core of our fifth point, this politico-cultural revamp of democracy can complement but not substitute for the overdue politico-legal reform of citizenship based on effective belonging. If anything, the COVID-19 pandemic has increased the polarizing effect on migrant populations between being called into 'effective membership' in times of crisis, but being more or less marginalized in terms of full citizenship in all its legal and cultural facets when the normal state of affairs resumes. Notions of 'multi-level citizenship' that go beyond local voting rights for non-nationals need to be further discussed in the light of the COVID-19 experience (Triandafyllidou, 2022; Bauböck, 2020).

The owl of Minerva only spreads its wings at dusk, when the contours of a past epoch stand out more clearly, we have learned from Hegel, the philosopher of world history. Has theCOVID-19 pandemic already passed, and if so, has it passed long enough for us to realize the contours of a post-pandemic society? Even historians are not quite sure whether a global assessment of this pandemic is 'too early' as yet, but they also maintain that 'it is never too soon to begin learning from your mistakes' (Ferguson, 2022, p. 397f.). Thus, the question whether the COVID-19 pandemic can eventually be compared with the 'Black Death' that reached Europe in the fourteenth century, implying that it has perhaps not caused but contributed to 'the patterns of several centuries [...] breaking up; not only the pattern of society but the set of men's [sic!] minds as well' (Ziegler, 1998/1969, p. 247), is a question of world historical dimension that we had better leave to the course of history and future historians. For the moment it would appear that COVID-19 might stand better comparison with the Asian flu of 1957/1958 in terms of the suspected Chinese origin, its eventual global spread and its impact—'a major crisis of global public health at the time, but fifty years later largely forgotten' (Ferguson, 2022, pp. 380, 215f.).

However, as far issues of integration and migration are concerned, the Spanish flu pandemic of 1918/1919 offers itself even better to comparison due to its intersection with a major wave of transatlantic migration (Boris, 2022, p. 66f.; Kraut, 2010). Here the historical report reveals striking similarities to COVID-19 and our research: the initial fear of 'pathogens arriving on the bodies of newcomers'; the stigmatization and scapegoating of the most vulnerable migrants that due to heteronormative custom (spitting, not using handkerchiefs) and lifestyle (large families in small accommodation and 'the desire to be close, not distant' in case of sickness) were thought to spread the disease—here notably Chinese as well as Italian migrants—the role of community leaders and native-born physicians as 'important mediators between public health officials and immigrants'; the importance of self-help infrastructures set up by migrant communities (starting from foreign language press as channels of relevant information and education, to migrants' churches as meeting places and even ethnic clinics as places of culturally sensitive care), to name but a few (Kraut, 2010).

Yet, there is one important discontinuity amidst all this seeming pandemic continuity that we should not overlook when considering COVID-19 today and in the future. COVID-19, more than any other pandemic, is tied up with other potential hazards and risks: from climate change and amoral AI, to real regional and potential world wars, all connected to mass migration. A potential COVID-23 or COVID-27 will not necessarily meet a better prepared world society but, quite possibly, one tied up in a highly disruptive complexity and a resulting dystopic world view (Ferguson, 2022, pp. 383–389). Historians maintain for the social transformation initiated by both the plague and the twentieth century flu pandemics an underlying sense of progress and optimism. With regard to the plague this reads: 'the Black Death did no more than accelerate, though often violently accelerate, an established, and in the long run, inevitable progress' (Ziegler 1998/1969, p. 252), while for the aftermath of the Asian flu, Ferguson (2022, p. 12) refers to 'a time of seeming progress'. Yet, the COVID-19 pandemic has met with a 'global epidemic of nostalgia', as Bauman (2017, p. 3) has aptly described the prevailing mental disposition of contemporary Western society. This means that 'the future is transformed from the natural habitat of hopes and rightful expectations into the site of nightmares' (ibid., p. 6). 'Retrotopia' is the place where the 'gap between power and politics—that is, the ability to have things done and the capacity to decide what things need to be done—[deepens]' (ib,: 12).

Still, as we have seen in the narratives with our interlocutors, this is not the time for intellectual depression or political inertia nor for civic freezing. The attitude prevailing amongst those keeping things running in times of crisis and in a world of latent nostalgia we would describe with Bardhan (2022, p. 5) as 'upbeat scepticism: pushing for things to get better while being aware that they may not'.

References

Albrow, M. (2014). Local Integrities and Global Interconnectedness. In M. Albrow (Ed.), *Global Age Essays on Social and Cultural Change* (pp. 127–137). Klostermann.

Appadurai, A., & Robles-Anderson, E. (2023). Solidarity's Fragilities. *Public Culture, 35*(1), 1–6. https://doi.org/10.1215/08992363-10202332

Bauböck, R. (2020). In Defence of Multilevel Citizenship—a Rejoinder. In R. Bauböck & L. Orgad (Eds.), *Cities vs. States: Should Urban Citzenship be Emancipated from Nationality?* (EUI Working Paper) (pp. 79–86). European University Institute.

Bardhan, P. (2022). *A World of Insecurity: Democratic Disenchantment in Rich and Poor Countries.* Harvard Univ. Press.

Bauman, Z. (2017). *Retrotopia.* Polity.

Beck, U. (1995). *Ecological Politics in an Age of Risk.* Polity.

Boris, E. (2022). Vulnerability and Resilience in the Covid-19 Crisis: Race, Gender, and Belonging. In A. Triandafyllidou (Ed.), *Migration and Pandemics* (IMISCOE Research Series) (pp. 65–84). https://doi.org/10.1007/978-3-030-81210-2_1

Charquero-Ballester, M., Walter, J. G., Nissen, I.A., & Bechmann, A. (2021, July–December). Different types of COVID-19 Misinformation Have Different Emotional Valence on Twitter. *Big Data & Society*, 1–11. https://doi.org/10.1177/20539517211041279.

Ferguson, N. (2022). *Doom: The Politics of Catastrophe.* Penguin UK.

Ferrarello, S. (2021). The Normative Spaces of Resilience. *Journal of Artificial Intelligence Humanities, 12/2*(24), 267–284.

Hartley, K., & Jarvis, D. S. L. (2020). Policymaking in a Low-trust state: Legitimacy, State Capacity, and Responses to COVID-19 in Hong Kong. *Policy and Society, 39*(3), 403–423.

Hochschild, A. R. (2018). *Strangers in Their Own Land: Anger and Mourning on the American Right.* The New Press.

Kraut, A. M. (2010). Immigration, Ethnicity, and the Pandemic. *Public Health Reports, 125*(3), 123–133.

Mu, G. M. (2021). Sociologising Resilience Through Bourdieu's Field Analysis: Misconceptualisation, Conceptualisation, and Reconceptualization. *British Journal of Sociology of Education, 42*(1), 15–31.

Obrist, B., Pfeiffer, C., & Hentley, R. (2010). Multi-layered Social Resilience: A New Approach in Mitigation Research. *Progress in Development Studies, 10*(4), 283–293.

Rosanvallon, P. (2014). *Das Parlament der Unsichtbaren*. Blinklicht.

Triandafyllidou, A. (2022). Spaces of Solidarity and Spaces of Exception: Migration and Membership During Pandemic Times. In A. Triandafyllidou (ed.), *Migration and Pandemics* (pp. 3–21), IMISCOE Research Series. https://doi.org/10.1007/978-3-030-81210-2_1

Ziegler, Ph. (1998/1969). *The Black Death*. Penguin.

Index[1]

[1] Note: Page numbers followed by 'n' refer to notes.

M. Caselli et al. (eds.), *Migrants' (Im)mobilities in Three European Urban Contexts*, Europe in a Global Context,
https://doi.org/10.1007/978-3-031-53773-8

SPRINGER NATURE

GPSR Compliance

The European Union's (EU) General Product Safety Regulation (GPSR) is a set of rules that requires consumer products to be safe and our obligations to ensure this.

If you have any concerns about our products, you can contact us on ProductSafety@springernature.com

In case Publisher is established outside the EU, the EU authorized representative is:

Springer Nature Customer Service Center GmbH
Europaplatz 3
69115 Heidelberg, Germany

FSC
www.fsc.org
MIX
Papier | Fördert gute Waldnutzung
FSC® C083411

Kolibri 360 GmbH
Ferdinand-Jühlke-Straße 7
99095 Erfurt, Deutschland
produktsicherheit@kolibri360.de